NURSING PHOTOBOOK™

Coping with Neurologic Disorders

NURSING82 BOOKS
INTERMED COMMUNICATIONS, INC.
SPRINGHOUSE, PENNSYLVANIA

NURSING82 BOOKS

NURSING PHOTOBOOK™ SERIES
Providing Respiratory Care
Managing I.V. Therapy
Dealing with Emergencies
Giving Medications
Assessing Your Patients
Using Monitors
Providing Early Mobility
Giving Cardiac Care
Performing GI Procedures
Implementing Urologic Procedures
Controlling Infection
Ensuring Intensive Care
Coping with Neurologic Disorders
Caring for Surgical Patients
Working with Orthopedic Patients
Nursing Pediatric Patients
Helping Geriatric Patients
Attending Ob/Gyn Patients
Aiding Ambulatory Patients
Carrying Out Special Procedures

NURSING SKILLBOOK® SERIES
Reading EKGs Correctly
Dealing with Death and Dying
Managing Diabetics Properly
Assessing Vital Functions Accurately
Helping Cancer Patients Effectively
Giving Cardiovascular Drugs Safely
Giving Emergency Care Competently
Monitoring Fluid and Electrolytes Precisely
Documenting Patient Care Responsibly
Combatting Cardiovascular Diseases Skillfully
Coping with Neurologic Problems Proficiently
Using Crisis Intervention Wisely
Nursing Critically Ill Patients Confidently

NURSE'S REFERENCE LIBRARY™
Diseases
Diagnostics

***Nursing81* DRUG HANDBOOK™**

PROFESSIONAL GUIDE TO DRUGS™

NURSING PHOTOBOOK™ Series
PUBLISHER
Eugene W. Jackson

EDITORIAL DIRECTOR
Jean Robinson

CLINICAL DIRECTOR
Barbara McVan, RN

ART DIRECTOR
Lisa A. Gilde

**Intermed Communications
Book Division**
DIRECTOR
Timothy B. King

DIRECTOR, RESEARCH
Elizabeth O'Brien

DIRECTOR, PRODUCTION AND PURCHASING
Bacil Guiley

Staff for this volume
BOOK EDITOR
Patricia R. Urosevich

CLINICAL EDITOR
Paulette J. Strauch, RN

ASSOCIATE EDITORS
Paul Vigna, Jr.
Richard Samuel West

PHOTOGRAPHER
Paul A. Cohen

ASSOCIATE DESIGNERS
Linda Jovinelly Franklin
Scott M. Stephens
Carol Stickles

DESIGN ASSISTANT
Darcy Moore Feralio

ASSISTANT PHOTOGRAPHER
Thomas Staudenmayer

EDITORIAL/GRAPHIC COORDINATOR
Doreen K. Stowers

CLINICAL/GRAPHIC COORDINATOR
Evelyn M. James

COPY EDITOR
Sharyl D. Wolf

EDITORIAL STAFF ASSISTANT
Cynthia A. O'Connell

PHOTOGRAPHY ASSISTANT
Frank Margeson

ART PRODUCTION MANAGER
Robert Perry

ARTISTS
Diane Fox   Joan Walsh
Sandra Simms   Robert Walsh
Louise Stamper   Ron Yablon

RESEARCHER
Vonda Heller

TYPOGRAPHY MANAGER
David C. Kosten

TYPOGRAPHY ASSISTANTS
Janice Auch Haber
Ethel Halle
Diane Paluba
Nancy Wirs

PRODUCTION MANAGERS
Wilbur D. Davidson
Robert L. Dean, Jr.

PRODUCTION ASSISTANT
Donald G. Knauss

ILLUSTRATORS
Art People Assoc.   Bob Jones
Dimitrios Bastas   Polly Krumbhaar Lewis
John Dougherty   Cynthia Mason
Jean Gardner   Dan Sneberger
Robert Jackson

SERIES GRAPHIC DESIGNER
John C. Isely

COVER PHOTO
Photographic Illustrations

**Clinical consultants
for this volume**

Rita T. Giubilato, RN, BSN, MSN
Staff Development Coordinator
Neurosensory Care Program
Thomas Jefferson University Hospital
Philadelphia, Pa.

Celestine B. Mason, RN, BSN, MA
Associate Professor
Pacific Lutheran University School of Nursing
Tacoma, Wash.

Copyright © 1981 by Intermed
Communications, Inc.,
1111 Bethlehem Pike, Springhouse, PA 19477
All rights reserved. Reproduction in
whole or part by any means
whatsoever without written permission
of the publisher is prohibited by law.
Printed in the United States of America.

011281

Library of Congress Cataloging in Publication Data

Main entry under title:

Coping with neurologic disorders.

  (Nursing photobook)
  "Nursing81 books."
  Bibliography: p.
  Includes index.
  1. Neurological nursing.   2. Neurologic examination.
I. Series. [DNLM: 1. Neurology—Atlases.   2. Neurology—
Nursing texts. WY 160 C783]
RC350.5.C658   616.8   81-13364
ISBN 0-916730-42-5   AACR2

Contents

Introduction

Reviewing neurologic basics

CONTRIBUTORS TO
THIS SECTION INCLUDE:
Rosemary Noone McCormick, RN, BSN
Connie A. Walleck, RN, CNRN, BSN, MS

Managing diagnostic procedures

CONTRIBUTORS TO
THIS SECTION INCLUDE:
Lester J. Gardina, RN, BS

Monitoring your patient

CONTRIBUTORS TO
THIS SECTION INCLUDE:
Susan E. Galada, RN, CNRN
Donna Ranieri-Ambrogi, RN

Dealing with neurologic problems

CONTRIBUTORS TO
THIS SECTION INCLUDE:
Rita T. Giubilato, RN, BSN, MSN
Frances W. Sills, RN, BSN, MSN
Paulette J. Strauch, RN

Fulfilling patient potential

CONTRIBUTORS TO
THIS SECTION INCLUDE:
Carol H . Best, RN, CNRN
Mary Pat Erdner, RN, BSN
Janet G. LaMantia, RN, BSN, MA
Maureen Quinn McKeown, RN, BSN, MA
Jerry Tupy, RN, ADN

Contributors

At the time of original publication, these contributors held the following positions.

Donna Ranieri-Ambrogi is a staff nurse in the neurological intensive care unit at the University of California's Moffitt Hospital in San Francisco. She holds a nursing diploma from Thomas Jefferson University Hospital School of Nursing and is a BSN degree candidate at the University of San Francisco. She is a member of the American Nurses' Association.

Carol H. Best, head nurse of the neurological intensive care unit at Barrow Neurological Institute, St. Joseph's Hospital and Medical Center, Phoenix, Arizona, has joined the NURSING PHOTOBOOK staff as a clinical editor. Ms. Best attended Villanova (Pa.) University for 2 years as a general nursing student, and earned a nursing diploma at Philadelphia General Hospital School of Nursing. A certified neurosurgical registered nurse, Ms. Best is a member of the American Association of Neurosurgical Nurses.

Mary Pat Erdner is assistant head nurse at Magee Memorial Hospital Rehabilitation Center in Philadelphia. She earned a BSN degree at Pennsylvania State University, University Park, Pennsylvania. Ms. Erdner is a member of the Pennsylvania Chapter of the Greater Delaware Valley District of the Association of Rehabilitation Nurses.

Susan E. Galada, a certified neurosurgical registered nurse, is a staff nurse in the central nervous system unit at Allentown (Pa.) and Sacred Heart Hospital Center. She has a nursing diploma from Allentown Hospital School of Nursing and was a student in Montreal Neurologic Institute's post-basic nursing program. Ms. Galada is a member of the American Association of Neurosurgical Nurses.

Lester J. Gardina is a head nurse at St. Joseph's Hospital and Medical Center, Phoenix, Arizona. He earned a nursing diploma at Phoenix (Ariz.) College, and he has a BS degree in business administration and management from Arizona State University, Tempe, Arizona. Mr. Gardina is a member of Arizona Nurses in Management.

Rita T. Giubilato, an advisor for this PHOTOBOOK, is staff development coordinator of the neurosensory care program at Thomas Jefferson University Hospital, Philadelphia. Ms. Giubilato holds a nursing diploma from the Hospital of the University of Pennsylvania School of Nursing, Philadelphia; a BSN degree from Seton Hall University, South Orange, New Jersey; and an MSN degree from Philadelphia's University of Pennsylvania. She is a member of the American Association of Neurosurgical Nurses, and the American Association of Critical-Care Nurses.

Janet G. LaMantia is clinical coordinator of the Regional Spinal Cord Injury Center of Delaware Valley, Thomas Jefferson University Hospital and Magee Memorial Hospital Rehabilitation Center. She earned a BSN degree at Hunter College, New York, and holds an MA degree from New York (N.Y.) University. Ms. LaMantia is a member of the Association of Rehabilitation Nurses, and the Pennsylvania Chapter of the Greater Delaware Valley District of the Association of Rehabilitation Nurses.

Rosemary Noone McCormick is charge nurse on a medical floor at Kirksville (Mo.) Osteopathic Hospital. She earned a BSN degree at Wilkes College, Wilkes-Barre, Pennsylvania. Ms. McCormick also completed a neurologic nursing internship program at Massachusetts General Hospital in Boston.

Maureen Quinn McKeown, assistant director of nursing at Magee Memorial Hospital Rehabilitation Center, Philadelphia, earned a nursing diploma at Suffolk School of Nursing, Southampton (N.Y.) Hospital. She has a BSN degree from Long Island University, Brooklyn (N.Y.) Center and an MA degree in rehabilitation nursing from New York (N.Y.) University. Ms. McKeown is a member of the America Congress of Physical Medicine and Rehabilitation; the Association of Rehabilitation Nurses; the Pennsylvania Chapter of the Greater Delaware Valley District of the Association of Rehabilitation Nurses; and Sigma Theta Tau.

Celestine B. Mason, an advisor for this PHOTOBOOK, is an associate professor at Pacific Lutheran University School of Nursing, Tacoma, Washington. She earned a BSN degree at the Catholic University of America in Washington, D.C. In addition, she has an MA degree from Pacific Lutheran University, Tacoma, Washington. Ms. Mason is coauthor of NEUROLOGIC CRITICAL CARE and holds memberships in the American Nurses' Association, the American Association of Critical-Care Nurses, and the American Association of Neurosurgical Nurses.

Frances W. Sills is director of nursing of the Ortho-Rehab-Neuro Hospital Center at James M. Jackson Memorial Hospital in Miami. She earned a nursing diploma at St.Mary's Hospital of Rochester (Minn.) School of Nursing. She holds a BSN degree from the University of Miami, Coral Gables, Florida, and an MSN degree from the University of Alabama, Tuscaloosa. Ms. Sills is a member of the American Nurses' Association, the Florida Nurses' Association, the American Nurses' Association, the Florida Nurses' Association, the American Association of Neurosurgical Nurses, and Sigma Theta Tau.

Jerry Tupy is a head nurse at Magee Memorial Hospital Rehabilitation Center, Philadelphia. He earned an associate's degree in nursing at Community College of Philadelphia and is a member of the Association of Rehabilitation Nurses. Mr. Tupy is also chairperson of the patient/family teaching committee at Magee Memorial Hospital Rehabilitation Center.

Connie A. Walleck is a nurse clinician II in the department of neurosurgery at University of Maryland Hospital, Baltimore. Ms. Walleck earned a nursing diploma at Presbyterian-University Hospital School of Nursing in Pittsburgh. She holds a BSN degree from the University of Maryland at Baltimore, and is an MS degree candidate there.

Introduction

What's your reaction when someone says neurologic disorder? Do you think of the time, patience, and expert nursing skills required to care for a patient with such a disorder? If you do, you have a good understanding of what's expected. Not only are many neurologic disorders irreversible, but the patient's physical condition may vary from minute to minute. In addition to assessing, monitoring, and providing nursing care, you must be ready to give emotional support to the patient and his family.

From hour to hour, the patient and his family will look to you for explanations, answers to their questions, and reassurance. That's why knowing as much as possible about neurologic nursing is essential. That's also why we've gone beyond the basics to offer you a PHOTOBOOK suited to the needs, special interests, and challenges that are part of neurologic nursing. This is the first book to take you step-by-step through 12 diagnostic testing procedures. And it puts how-to photos, illustrations, charts, and information-packed text at your fingertips.

To help you better understand the underlying causes of neurologic disorders, we've opened this PHOTOBOOK with a review of neurologic anatomy and physiology.

Next, we take you through a complete neurologic assessment. In it, we'll show you how to test your patient's tactile discrimination, how to perform the Romberg test, and how to check for the Babinski response. We'll also tell you how to interpret the results of these tests.

Knowing how to properly monitor a patient with a neurologic disorder is critical, because his condition may change at any time. If you follow the information contained in Section 3, you'll learn how. For example, we'll show you how to interpret pupillary reactions and evaluate respiratory patterns. You'll also see how to perform an hour-to-hour neurocheck. But that's not all.

We'll also show you how to: perform a neurocheck at the scene of an accident; use a computerized neurocheck sheet; and differentiate intracranial pressure monitoring systems. In another section of this book, we discuss neurologic disorders—how to recognize the signs and symptoms, and what complications to expect. We'll tell you how to provide complete and competent care for a patient with such a disorder. But sooner or later your patient with a neurologic disorder will return home. To help make this transition go smoothly, we detail how to help your patient and his family compensate and live with a neurologic deficit; be it respiratory, bowel, bladder, or sexual.

COPING WITH NEUROLOGIC DISORDERS gives you more options and more alternatives on the way you care for your patient. This PHOTOBOOK may even help you save his life.

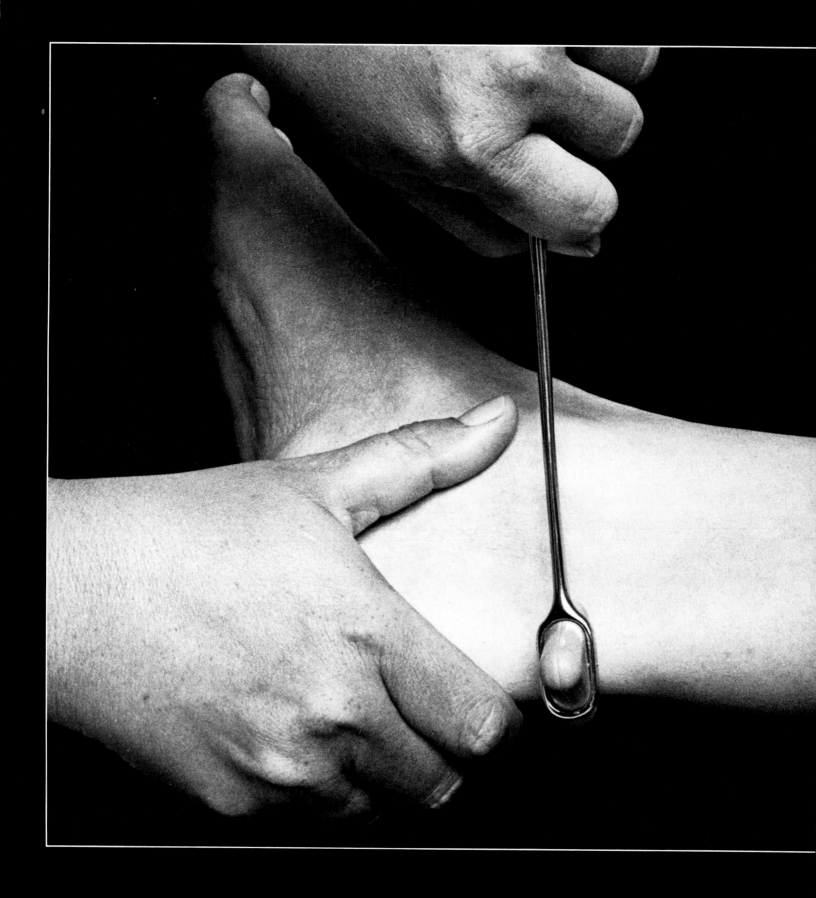

Reviewing Neurologic Basics

Anatomy and physiology

Assessment

Anatomy and physiology

"Isn't there anyone around here who can tell me what's wrong with me?" shouts 43-year-old Tom Boyle. Mr. Boyle's upset. He's just been admitted to your unit with a suspected space-occupying brain lesion.

"What's a space-occupying lesion?" he demands. "Does it mean I'm going to die?" As you look around Mr. Boyle's room, you spot Mrs. Boyle wringing her hands. She tells you she's also worried her husband will die, or at best need surgery, become an invalid, and lose his job.

What can you do? As a nurse, you can help the couple understand Mr. Boyle's suspected condition. But first, thoroughly review what you know about neurologic anatomy and physiology.

Then, take the time to describe normal brain structure and function to Mr. Boyle. Explain what a space-occupying lesion is and how it causes his signs and symptoms.

Read carefully the pages that follow. If you always keep in mind how a normal neurologic system functions, you'll be better able to understand and help your patient understand his neurologic disorder.

Differentiating neurons and glia cells

The nervous system is probably the most complicated and delicately balanced system in the body. When something happens to upset that balance—for example, trauma, infection, or disease—the result may be devastating.

To understand the nervous system completely, start with the most basic unit: the cell.

A closer look at cells

As you know, two major cell types make up the nervous system: neurons or nerve cells which receive and transmit messages; and glia cells (collectively called neuroglia) which support and protect the neurons. Glia cells are nonexcitable.

Neurons: Neurons come in a variety of shapes and sizes, depending on their location and function in the nervous system.

But, when we talk about neurologic disorders, we're referring to the abnormal functioning of three basic neuron types: motor, sensory, and internuncial. These three neuron types conduct impulses toward and away from the central nervous system (CNS) and transmit impulses from nerve center to nerve center within the CNS.

Regardless of its type, though, each neuron has short twiglike projections called *dendrites* that receive impulses from adjacent cells and relay them to the cell body. Within the cell body is a nucleus which conducts complex chemical reactions that keep the cell alive and functioning.

The axon, on the other hand, is a long projection—sometimes greater than 24" (61 cm)—which transmits impulses away from the cell body. This axon may contact an adjacent neuron directly, contact neighboring dendrites, or terminate at the affected organ.

Of course, a white fatty substance, called myelin, covers most larger neurons. Myelin insulates neurons, allowing impulses to travel more smoothly and quickly. Myelinated neurons make up the cranial and spinal nerves and are located in the white matter of the brain and spinal cord.

A sheath of Schwann's cells, commonly called neurilemma, envelops cells outside the CNS, aiding myelin formation. And, if the axon's cut or injured, neurilemma stimulates axon regeneration. But remember, neurons inside the CNS are not covered with neurilemma, and therefore, are incapable of regeneration.

Glia cells: Besides their protective and supportive characteristics, glia cells are known for one other distinguishing trait: rapid reproduction. Unlike neurons, glia cells divide by mitosis and quickly produce daughter cells. In fact, glia cells make up the majority of cells in the nervous system.

Is all this important to neurologic disorders? Yes. Because a patient exhibiting signs and symptoms of a brain tumor actually has a neuroglia overgrowth. In this case, glia cells reproduce faster than the available space, creating pain, and pressure on vital brain parts, which demands medical attention. With or without treatment, neuroglia growths may be fatal.

Understanding the brain's anatomy

When you envision the human cranium, think of a semi-circular mass with a hard fibrous outer coating. As you'll remember, the cranium protects and houses the brain and nervous system. That's why understanding cranial anatomy is so important.

Let's first review the cranium's major bones, which are labeled by the portion of brain that they cover: frontal, parietal, temporal, and occipital. Immovable joints called sutures unite the cranial bones.

Now keep in mind that the brain is enveloped by three meninges called the dura mater, arachnoid, and the pia mater. These meninges also cover the spinal cord.

Portions of the dura mater—the falx cerebri and the tentorium—extend into the brain's fissures. The falx cerebri lies in the longitudinal fissure, and separates the right and left hemispheres. The tentorium lies in the transverse fissure and separates the cerebrum and cerebellum.

As you can see in this illustration, a narrow channel called the subdural space separates the dura mater from the arachnoid. A second channel, called the subarachnoid space, lies between the arachnoid and the pia mater. (Cerebrospinal fluid [CSF] and the brain's larger blood vessels are contained within the subarachnoid space.)

You'll remember that the cranium's numerous openings, or foramina, permit nerves and blood vessels to exit and enter the brain. These foramina, located in the subarachnoid area, allow CSF to circulate through the spinal cord and brain.

Each of the brain's four ventricles contains a cluster of capillaries, called the choroid plexus. These capillaries produce CSF. From the ventricles, CSF circulates through the brain and spinal cord, cushioning it from injury and transporting wastes and nutrients. At any given time, 100 to 150 ml of CSF is circulating through a healthy adult. Eventually, the brain's venous sinus—primarily the superior saggital sinus—absorbs the CSF through the arachnoid villi.

Look again at the illustration. You'll see two of the larger foramina, the tentorial notch, and foramen magnum. If a patient's brain is injured, the resulting edema may cause brain tissue to herniate through one of these large foramina. This condition, known as tentorial herniation, is usually fatal.

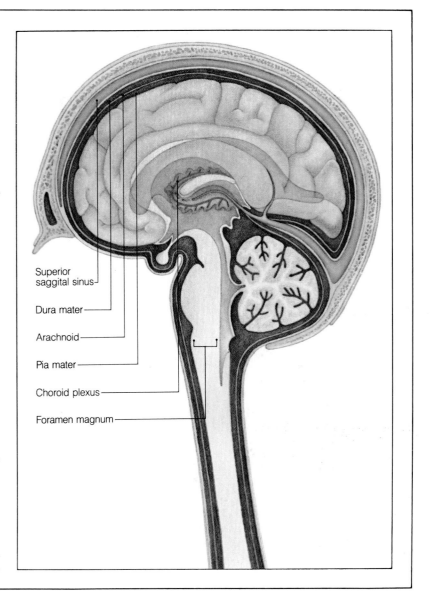

Superior saggital sinus

Dura mater

Arachnoid

Pia mater

Choroid plexus

Foramen magnum

What's a neuron?

Reviewing neurologic basics? If so, you'll probably start with the most basic brain unit: the nerve cell or neuron. While neurons have many different functions, their main job is to receive and transmit impulses. But did you know:
* more than 10 billion neurons make up the brain?
* neurons release chemicals which transmit information from one neuron to another?
* neurons in the brain's cortex affect what you do, feel, and think?

Remember that disease, trauma, or drugs may affect normal neuron functioning. In some cases, abnormally functioning neurons cause neurologic disorders. Do you know which ones cause which disorders?
* Input neurons cause hallucinations.
* Processing neurons cause memory loss, under or overreaction to emotional situations, clouded judgment, fainting spells, or coma.
* Output neurons cause loss of muscular coordination; muscle paralysis in arms, legs, and other body parts; and epilepsy.

Anatomy and physiology

Learning about the brain

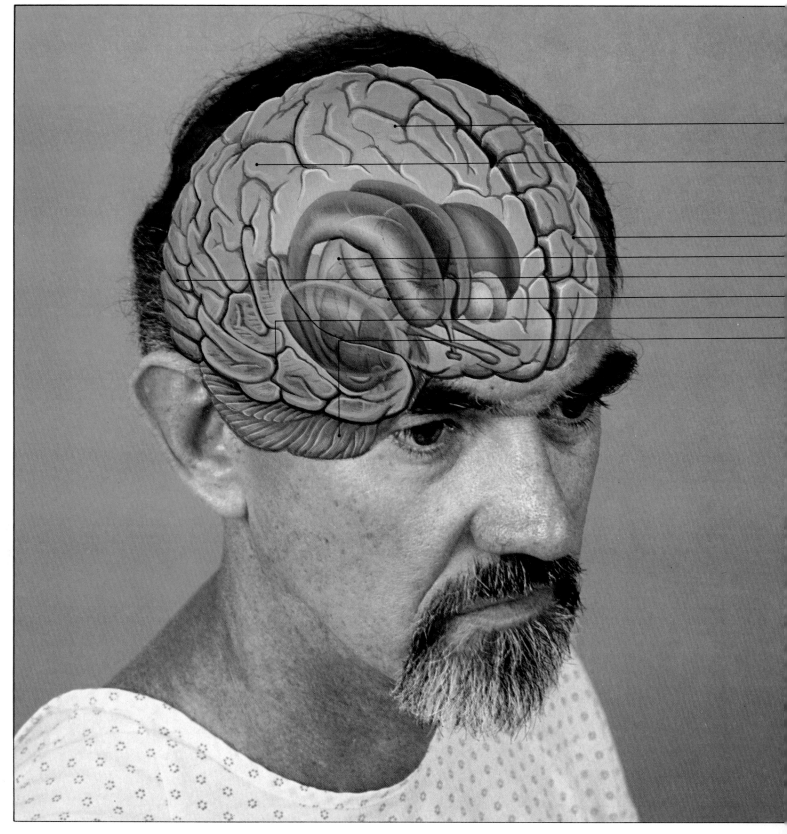

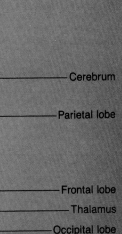

Cerebrum

Parietal lobe

Frontal lobe

Thalamus

Occipital lobe

Midbrain

Temporal lobe

Cerebellum

Entering a patient's brain is like opening the door to a complex control panel. Not only does the brain control how a patient adapts to his environment, it also affects what he does and says.

Obviously a finely tuned mass of membrane, tissue, and fluid, the brain is the center of emotions, thoughts, and feelings. It coordinates, channels, and controls the body. It's the basis for all behavior.

Simply speaking, we'll say the brain is composed of the cerebrum, cerebellum, and brain stem. These parts, and many others, form the nervous system.

As you'll remember, the nervous system has three divisions: the central nervous system, consisting of the brain and spinal cord; the peripheral nervous system, containing nerves extending throughout the body; for example, cranial and spinal nerves; and the autonomic nervous system, consisting of the sympathetic and parasympathetic systems.

Now, read on to find out more about the brain's components.

CEREBRUM
Sitting on top of the spinal cord above the cerebellum, the cerebrum is contained in the anterior and middle cranial fossae. The cerebrum is the brain's largest part. As you know, a longitudinal fissure divides the cerebrum into two halves: the right and left hemispheres. In addition, a broad band of white connecting fiber, called the *corpus callosum,* joins both hemispheres at the fissure's base. This band allows communication between the hemispheres.

The convoluted outer surface of each hemisphere is interspersed with furrows commonly called *sulci.*

Each hemisphere consists of an outer layer of gray matter composed of unmyelinated neurons, (which contains a cerebral cortex, and basal ganglia nuclei); and an inner core of white matter containing myelinated axons.

Most of the brain's higher mental activities, such as memory and reasoning, are centered in the cerebral cortex. Why? Because the cortex receives and evaluates impulses, receives and stockpiles intelligence, and controls voluntary movements.

Within the cerebrum's gray matter is the nuclei of the thalamus, which relays sensations such as touch, pain, hot, and cold; the hypothalamus, which governs appetite, body temperature, sleep, and emotions, such as anger and fear; and the basal ganglia, which inhibit excessive movement and lend smoothness to cerebral cortical actions. Even the most minute stimulation of the thalamus, hypothalamus, or basal ganglia fires nerve cells—like a string of firecrackers—until the message reaches the cortex.

On the other hand, the cerebrum's white matter is made up of myelinated nerve fibers. And these fibers connect the cortex, brain, and spinal cord.

Sulci, which we already described, separate the cerebrum's hemispheres into four lobes: frontal, parietal, temporal, and occipital. Each lobe contains separate controls for basic brain function, as follows.

Remember: Each cerebral hemisphere works principally with one side of the body. A lesion in one hemisphere presents signs and symptoms on the opposite side of the body.

FRONTAL LOBE
• *Prefrontal area* partially controls respirations, gastrointestinal activity, circulation, pupillary reactions, and emotion. In addition, this area helps regulate personality, thought processes, intellect, conceptualization, mathematical abilities, and concentration.
• *Broca's motor speech area* controls ability to articulate speech. This area is contained in one hemisphere and is almost always dominant in the left hemisphere. Damage to this area may cause motor aphasia.
• *Written speech area* controls the ability to write words. As you know, right- or left-handedness is partially governed by cerebral dominance. But no matter whether a patient is right- or left-handed, the written and spoken speech areas are usually situated in the left cerebral cortex.

TEMPORAL LOBE
• *Auditory speech area* integrates sound stimulus into pitch, quality, and loudness. It also identifies and integrates sounds with past experiences (long-term auditory memory).

PARIETAL LOBE
• *Wernicke's area* works in conjunction with the temporal lobe in understanding and interpreting a spoken word and written language. However, most of this activity is contained in the dominant cerebral hemisphere.
• *Postcentral area* receives stimulation from the spinal cord and controls the body's sensory areas.
• *Speech area of patient's dominant hemisphere* receives and interprets sensory impulses from the skin, muscle, tendons, joints, and mucous membranes. It also provides ability to perceive and discriminate by touch; for example, two-point discrimination.

OCCIPITAL LOBE
• *Visual sensory area* integrates visual stimulation for size, form, motion, and color. Additionally, the area identifies, integrates, and associates visual images with past experiences (long term visual memory).

CEREBELLUM
The next largest section of the brain is the cerebellum. It's located beneath and at the back of the brain, between the occipital lobes of the cerebrum and brain stem. Like the cerebrum, the cerebellum is divided into two hemispheres, each composed of gray and white matter. As you probably know, the cerebellum governs walking, balance coordination, and muscular memory involved in habitual actions. But remember, voluntary movements are possible without the help of the cerebellum. However, these movements will appear clumsy and disorganized.

Remember: A lesion in a cerebellum hemisphere presents signs and symptoms on the same side of the body.

Anatomy and physiology

**Learning how the
cerebral vascular system works**

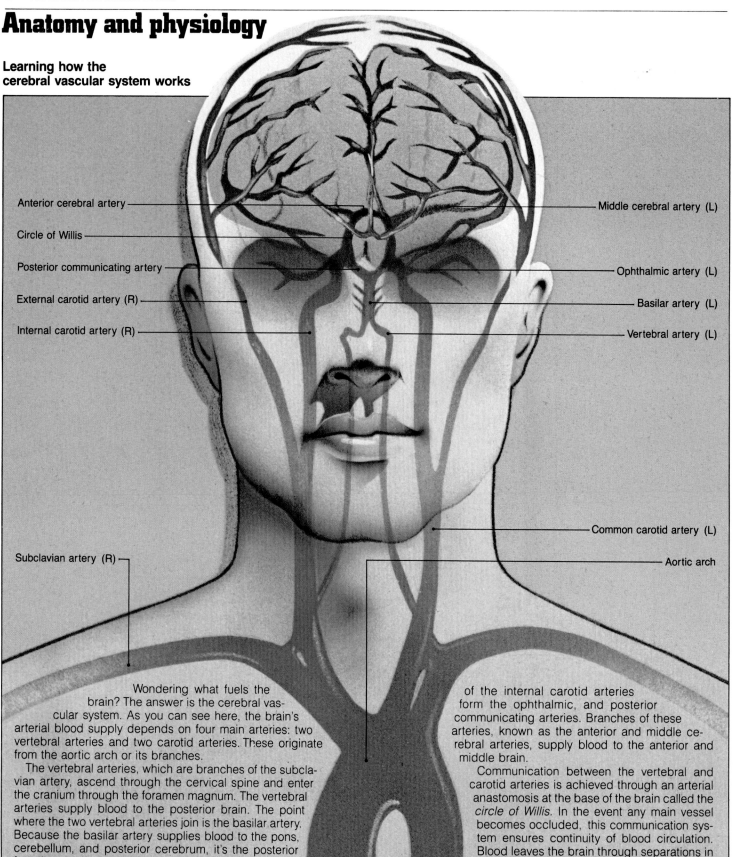

Anterior cerebral artery

Circle of Willis

Posterior communicating artery

External carotid artery (R)

Internal carotid artery (R)

Middle cerebral artery (L)

Ophthalmic artery (L)

Basilar artery (L)

Vertebral artery (L)

Common carotid artery (L)

Subclavian artery (R)

Aortic arch

Wondering what fuels the brain? The answer is the cerebral vascular system. As you can see here, the brain's arterial blood supply depends on four main arteries: two vertebral arteries and two carotid arteries. These originate from the aortic arch or its branches.

The vertebral arteries, which are branches of the subclavian artery, ascend through the cervical spine and enter the cranium through the foramen magnum. The vertebral arteries supply blood to the posterior brain. The point where the two vertebral arteries join is the basilar artery. Because the basilar artery supplies blood to the pons, cerebellum, and posterior cerebrum, it's the posterior fossa's most important artery.

As you probably know, the internal carotid arteries are branches of the common carotid arteries. And branches of the internal carotid arteries form the ophthalmic, and posterior communicating arteries. Branches of these arteries, known as the anterior and middle cerebral arteries, supply blood to the anterior and middle brain.

Communication between the vertebral and carotid arteries is achieved through an arterial anastomosis at the base of the brain called the *circle of Willis*. In the event any main vessel becomes occluded, this communication system ensures continuity of blood circulation. Blood leaves the brain through separations in the dura mater layers called sinuses. Larger sinuses follow courses made by fissures and ultimately drain into jugular veins.

Inside the brain stem: the medulla oblongata, pons, and midbrain

This illustration will help you visualize the brain stem and understand the importance of its parts: the medulla oblongata, pons, and midbrain.

For example, did you know that the medulla oblongata is the center of the body's respiratory system? Measuring about 1″ (2.5 cm), and situated just above the spinal cord, this area controls life-supporting reflexes such as breathing, gagging, coughing, swallowing, and articulating. Additionally, this area houses nuclei and motor components for several cranial nerves. The medulla oblongata, along with the thalamus and hypothalamus, integrates a network of nerve fibers making up the reticular activating system, which works as an arousal or alerting mechanism.

The pons, located between the midbrain and medulla oblongata, contains fiber tracts which enter and leave the brain. In addition, the pons contains nuclei and motor components of cranial nerves.

The portion of the cerebrum between the pons and diencephalon (consisting of the hypothalamus and thalamencephalon), is the midbrain. As you know, the midbrain conducts and relays impulses between higher and lower centers. Through the center of the midbrain runs a long tubular structure called the cerebral aqueduct or aqueduct of Sylvius, which carries cerebrospinal fluid between the third and fourth ventricles. The midbrain also houses nuclei for the cranial nerves.

Identifying the cranial nerves

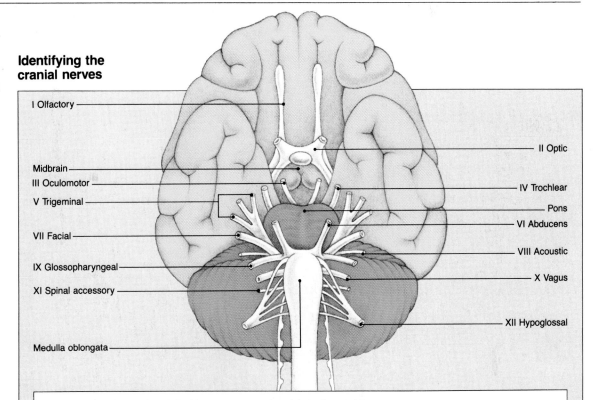

The midbrain, pons, and medulla oblongata serve as the origin for the cranial nerves.

As you know, cranial nerves transmit sensation from the body to the spinal cord and brain. They also transmit impulses from the brain and spinal cord to the body's muscles.

The 12 pairs of cranial nerves, along with the 31 pairs of spinal nerves, make up the peripheral nervous system. This system contains nerves which extend away from the central nervous system to the various parts of the body. And remember, cranial nerves innervate the same side of the body they originate on.

To recognize nerve complications, study the chart below. You'll find details on cranial nerve testing in the next section.

Nerve	Type	Function
I Olfactory	Sensory	Smell
II Optic	Sensory	Vision
III Oculomotor	Motor and sensory	Extraocular eye movement (up, down, and medial); pupillary constriction; upper lid elevation
IV Trochlear	Motor	Extraocular eye movement, including downward and lateral movements
V Trigeminal	Motor	Chewing, biting, and lateral jaw movements
VI Abducens	Motor	Face, scalp, teeth, and jaw sensation
	Sensory	Extraocular eye movement, including lateral eye movements
VII Facial	Motor	Facial muscles around eyes, mouth, and forehead
	Sensory	Taste receptors (anterior two thirds of tongue); salivary and lacrimal glands
VIII Acoustic	Sensory	Hearing; sense of balance
IX Glossopharyngeal	Motor	Secretion of saliva; swallowing movements
	Sensory	Sensations of throat; taste receptors (posterior one third of tongue)
X Vagus	Motor and sensory	Swallowing movement; voice production
XI Spinal accessory	Motor	Shoulder movements; neck rotation; nodding
XII Hypoglossal	Motor	Tongue movement

Important: The third, fourth, and sixth cranial nerves control all extraocular eye movements and their function will be tested together. Similarly, you will test the ninth, tenth, and twelfth cranial nerves when you evaluate the patient's ability to speak.

Anatomy and physiology

Looking at the spinal cord

When you're caring for a patient with signs of motor or sensory deficits, understanding the cord's structure and function becomes *crucial*.

A long cylindrical tube surrounded and protected by the vertebral column, the spinal cord's actually an extension of the medulla oblongata. Beginning at the foramen magnum, the spinal cord usually extends to the twelfth thoracic vertebra, but may continue as far as the second lumbar vertebra.

Like the brain, it's covered with protective layers called the dura mater, arachnoid mater, and pia mater.

For a closer look at the spinal cord, study the cross-section shown below. As you can see, the spinal cord's gray matter forms an H-shape and is surrounded by white matter.

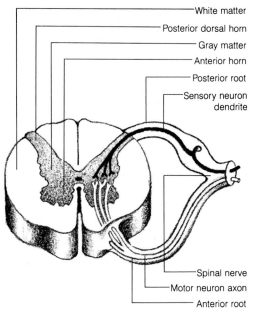

White matter
Posterior dorsal horn
Gray matter
Anterior horn
Posterior root
Sensory neuron dendrite
Spinal nerve
Motor neuron axon
Anterior root

A small oval-shaped canal filled with white matter is at the center of the gray matter and runs the entire length of the

spinal cord. The posterior dorsal portion of the gray H, also called the dorsal horn, relays sensory impulses from the body to the central nervous system (CNS). Cell bodies in the anterior or ventral horn relay motor impulses from the CNS to the skeletal muscles in the body's periphery.

Within the white matter are thousands of myelinated nerve fibers which form several tracts: the sensory (ascending) tract contains fibers running from the spinal cord to the brain; and the motor (descending) tracts contain fibers running from parts of the brain to the spinal cord.

You'll remember that the spinal cord has two functions: serving as the central trunk for conducting and relaying messages to and from the brain, and acting as a relay station between extremities and organs, and the brain.

But, besides conducting and relaying responsibilities, the spinal cord is also the body's most important reflex center. For example, when you tap your patient's elbow with a reflex hammer, you trigger a sensory impulse which travels to the spinal cord. The sensory impulse synapses with a motor neuron in the same cell in the same spinal cord segment. The outgoing motor impulse causes the elbow to withdraw.

So when a patient suffers spinal nerve damage, anterior or ventral nerve fibers and posterior or dorsal nerve fibers at the injury level become disconnected from nerve fibers above the injury level. Motor nerve fibers no longer transmit messages to muscles and glands; and sensory nerve fibers no longer transmit messages to tactile and discriminatory sensory nerve centers. In other words, all muscles, joints, tendons, organs, and sensory nerves at the injury level have a break in their relay station, and as a result, no longer function.

But remember, when a patient suffers a spinal cord injury, he'll experience upper motor neuron impairment at and below the injury level.

Identifying spinal nerves

Your patient's spinal nerves critically affect his ability to perceive and maneuver. These nerves are part of the peripheral nervous system. They originate in the spinal cord and leave the vertebral column through the intervertebral foramina.

As you probably know, the 31 pairs of spinal nerves are named by letter and number according to their exit point on the

spinal cord. Here's how they're distributed:
• eight pairs of cervical spinal nerves, C_1 to C_8
• twelve pairs of thoracic spinal nerves, T_1 to T_{12}
• five pairs of lumbar spinal nerves, L_1 to L_5
• five pairs of sacral spinal nerves, S_1 to S_5
• one pair of coccygeal spinal nerves.

Learning about the autonomic nervous system (ANS)

All bodily functions that happen automatically—without thought—are regulated by the autonomic nervous system (ANS). The ANS is also associated with emotional responses in stressful or high energy situations.

Composed of sensory and motor nerves, the ANS keeps the body functioning harmoniously by transmitting messages to involuntary or smooth muscles in organs such as the heart and bladder; glands such as the lacrimal and salivary; and to pupils, controlling size.

The ANS is divided into the sympathetic and parasympathetic systems.

Most organs have a double set of nerve fibers, one coming from the sympathetic system, and one from the parasympathetic system. Impulses from the sympathetic and parasympathetic systems have antagonistic effects.

The sympathetic system regulates the body's expenditure of energy, especially in times of stress. The parasympathetic system regulates bodily functions in everyday situations.

Wondering how the ANS works? Nerve cell bodies for the sympathetic system are located in the part of the spinal cord that runs through the thoracic and lumbar regions. Impulses from the central nervous system (CNS) reach these nerve cell bodies and travel along preganglionic nerve fibers.

In turn, these fibers run to a relay station called ganglion. From there, postganglionic nerve fibers proceed to their destination where they release catecholamine—*norepinephrine*. A form of adrenalin, norepinephrine transmits impulses across the synapses and junctions, accelerating body functions.

Nerve cell bodies in the parasympathetic system are situated in the extreme ends of the spinal cord—cranium or sacrum. Similar to sympathetic nerve fibers, they also transmit impulses from the CNS along preganglionic nerve fibers. But remember, their relay stations are positioned in or near the organ involved. These postganglionic fibers stimulate neurohormone release; *acetylcholine,* which acts as a neurotransmitter slowing body processes, and conserving body resources.

So the release of norepinephrine and acetylcholine by the sympathetic and parasympathetic systems depends on the body's immediate need to maintain or restore balance. So, the body's need determines the chemical amount to be released.

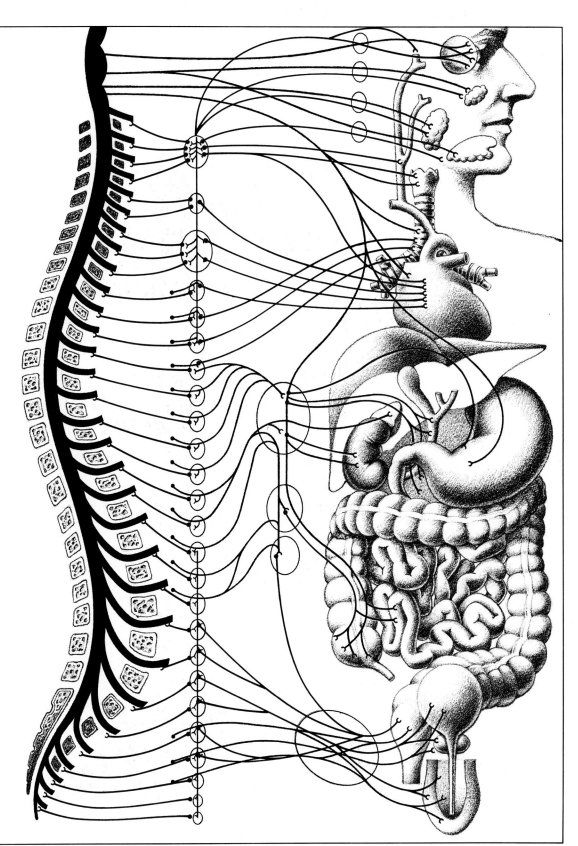

Nurses' guide to autonomic nervous system reactions

To keep the body functioning smoothly in both everyday situations and emotional crises, the sympathetic (see black lines) and parasympathetic (see red lines) systems of the autonomic nervous system (ANS) work hand in hand. Familiarize yourself with some of the more common effects the ANS has on the body, by reading this chart.

PUPIL
Sympathetic
Dilates
Parasympathetic
Constricts

SALIVARY GLAND
Sympathetic
Causes thick, viscous secretion
Parasympathetic
Causes watery secretion

BRONCHI
Sympathetic
Dilates
Parasympathetic
Constricts

HEART
Sympathetic
Increases rate
Parasympathetic
Decreases rate

CORONARY VESSELS
Sympathetic
Dilates
Parasympathetic
Causes no significant effect

GASTROINTESTINAL MUSCLE
Sympathetic
Inhibits peristalsis, stimulates sphincters
Parasympathetic
Stimulates peristalsis, inhibits sphincters

BLADDER
Sympathetic
Acts cooperatively with parasympathetic system in voiding
Parasympathetic
Contracts bladder muscle, relaxes sphincter

PENIS
Sympathetic
Causes ejaculation
Parasympathetic
Causes erection

SKELETAL MUSCLE VESSELS
Sympathetic
Constricts
Parasympathetic
Dilates

SKIN AND MOST OTHER VESSELS
Sympathetic
Constricts
Parasympathetic
Causes no significant effect

Assessment

In the last section, we reviewed how the neurologic system works. But do you know how to recognize and evaluate changes in it?

Consider the case of Mr. Boyle, who was recently admitted with a suspected space-occupying brain lesion. His signs and symptoms include vertigo, syncope, nausea, and seizures.

To form a data baseline that will help you and the doctor evaluate changes in Mr. Boyle's condition, you'll need to perform a thorough assessment, including a complete neurologic examination.

In the following pages, we'll show you how to:
• compile a thorough medical history (past and present), making sure you include information about your patient's family, any medications he's taking, and any allergies he has.
• assess your patient's emotional and mental status.
• conduct a thorough examination of your patient's nervous system by testing his cranial nerves, sensory system, motor function, and reflexes.

Performing a general assessment

Performing a thorough assessment of a patient with a suspected neurologic disorder is an essential and continual part of your nursing responsibility. You'll need to observe, evaluate, and document your patient's condition from the moment he enters your unit until he's discharged.

What constitutes a general assessment? It varies from hospital to hospital. But most likely, you'll need to obtain a thorough patient history, observe and evaluate your patient's emotional and mental status, and take his vital signs. Putting this information together allows you to evaluate your patient's overall health status, as well as any neurologic deficits he may have.

An equally important part of the assessment process is thorough and accurate documentation. Serving as a data baseline, this information will help you and the doctor identify any changes (for better or worse) in your patient's condition. As a result, you'll be able to adequately monitor your patient and provide better care.

Before beginning the general assessment, try to put him at ease by spending a few minutes talking with him. Make him as comfortable as possible; for example, elevate the head of his bed (if his condition permits). Be certain he can hear and understand you. Then, explain the purpose of the assessment and how the information will help you formulate his patient-care plan.

History taking

A carefully obtained history may provide your first clues to a possible neurologic disorder. Begin by finding out why your patient was admitted to the hospital. Try to elicit as much information as possible about what he thinks is the problem. Then, in easy to understand terms, ask him about specific signs and symptoms, using these questions as guidelines:
• Do you ever have blackout spells or dizziness? If so, how often do they occur and how long do they last? Do you ever hear loud noises or ringing in your ears prior to these spells?
• Do you vomit or feel nauseated frequently? If so, when does this occur? Do you vomit forcefully?
• Do you ever lose your balance? For example, as you walk, do you ever bump into people or lean against a wall for support?
• After sitting for a prolonged period of time, do you feel tingling or numbness?
• Do you ever cut or burn yourself without knowing it?
• Do you ever have headaches? If so, where do they occur? Are they dull, severe, or sharp? Do you take medication for them? If so, what do you take, and how often? Does the medication relieve the pain?
• Do you ever have seizures? If so, describe the seizure. Have you ever been diagnosed as having epilepsy? Do you take medication for either condition? If so, what do you take and how often?
• Are you currently under a doctor's care? Have you ever been treated by a neurosurgeon? If so, for what reason?

Next, ask your patient about any past illnesses, injuries, surgical procedures, and other medical or emotional conditions. If possible, include the diagnosis, dates, and any complications.

The patient's family history may reveal hereditary aspects of your patient's disorder. Note any familial diseases or conditions that may affect his nervous system, such as high blood pressure. Record the cause of death of any family member. Also, include your patient's marital status and whether he has any children. Occasionally, family situations such as divorce may induce emotional problems which present signs and symptoms similar to those of a neurologic disorder.

Finally, ask your patient if he has any allergies. Also, find out if he's taking any medications, including over-the-counter drugs. As you know, the side effects of some medications may cause or mask symptoms of a neurologic disorder. If he's taking medication, does he know what he's taking, why, and how often? If he doesn't know the name of the drug, he may be able to help you identify it by describing its color and shape. Has he ever stopped taking any of his medication without a doctor's order? If so, why?

Mental evaluation

As you take your patient's history, observe and evaluate him closely for clues about his emotional and mental status.

Watch his face as you interview him. Does he appear alert and attentive to your questioning? Does he make eye contact with you when you ask him a question or call his name? Or does he seem dull and drowsy, and stares into space? A lack of facial expression (also referred to as a flat affect) may indicate preoccupation, mental illness, drug abuse, subnormal intelligence or facial paralysis.

How would you describe his expression: confused, angry, impatient? Restlessness and irritability may indicate increased pain or intracranial pressure.

Observe your patient's facial expression. Does one eyelid droop slightly? Ptosis may indicate facial paralysis, myasthenia gravis, or tic douloureux. Does he twitch?

Your patient's appearance and behavior may also help identify a disorder. Observe him closely and ask yourself the following questions:
• What's his overall appearance? Is he clean and well-groomed? Or, does he appear disheveled? Observe his skin color. Is it jaundiced or flushed? If your patient's female, observe how she's applied her cosmetics (if she uses them). Are they applied incorrectly? For exam-

ple, is the lipstick too far above her lips? If so, she may have impaired vision, a perception problem, or tremors, indicating a possible neurologic disorder.
• When he speaks, does he have difficulty articulating? Does he lose his train of thought when answering questions? Are his responses clear and understandable, or are they garbled? Is he easily distracted? Subtle personality changes while speaking may be a sign of increased intracranial pressure or a tumor.

Note: Some disorders may be caused by paralysis.
• As your patient sits, observe his arms and legs. Does he have any paralysis? Does he appear relaxed, or does he make constant movements, such as pill-rolling his fingers, an indication of parkinsonism?
• Do his moods seem flighty, going from one extreme to the other? Does he exhibit any unusual mannerisms or reactions, such as sudden outbursts, uncontrollable crying or inappropriate laughter? Feelings of unreality, such as anger, fear, detachment, and deja vú may indicate psychomotor seizures.

To further assess your patient's neurologic condition, test his intellectual performance, which includes memory, orientation, and abstract reasoning. As you do, consider your patient's education and socioeconomic background.

While taking your patient's history, you've already assessed his long-term memory through his recollection of past events.

To test his short-term memory, tell him a short phrase or proverb, and ask him to repeat it 5 minutes later. Or, ask him to repeat a series of numbers. Has he noticed any change in his ability to remember things? If so, ask him to give an example.

Assess his orientation by asking him the date, time, and place. To assess his abstract reasoning, have him explain a simple proverb; for example, people in glass houses shouldn't throw stones.

Neurologic exam: checking vital signs

Whether your patient's conscious or unconscious, no assessment's complete without checking vital signs, including respiratory rate, blood pressure, pulse rate, and temperature. After establishing a baseline, changes in any of these vital signs may indicate a neurologic disorder. But that's not where your vital sign check ends. Here are some additional assessment points to keep in mind:
• Palpate all major arteries for pulsating masses and auscultate for bruits. Also check bilateral blood pressures and bilateral, major arterial pulses. Increased blood pressure and a decreased pulse rate may be signs of increased intracranial pressure.
• Check body temperature. Increased temperature may indicate damage to your patient's hypothalamus (the body's temperature-regulating center), or infection.
• Palpate the scalp. Soft scalp areas may indicate depressed skull fractures.
• Check cranial openings, such as nostrils and ear canals. Evidence of blood or spinal fluid drainage may indicate a skull fracture or a subdural hematoma.
• Assess your patient's respiratory system. An altered respiratory rate and pattern may signal existence or location of a lesion.
• Examine the torso and extremities. Look for bruises, hematomas, or lacerations which may indicate serious injury. Also check for fractures.

Document your findings in your nurses' notes.

Determining level of consciousness

As you know, level of consciousness refers to the degree your patient responds to stimuli and manipulations. Besides being a vital part of the neurologic exam, the patient's level of consciousness (when documented properly), is an effective indicator of his brain's functioning ability.

For example, an alert patient oriented to time, place, and person will respond appropriately to various stimuli (auditory, tactile, and visual). But when a patient's consciousness is impaired, evaluating and defining consciousness levels becomes difficult. Why? Because terms used to describe consciousness levels vary from hospital to hospital, and from health care professional to health care professional. Use the mini-assessment below when evaluating your patient's consciousness level. But remember, because no universally acceptable consciousness definitions exist, always document in detail your patient's response to all stimuli.

MINI-ASSESSMENT

 What's your patient's level of consciousness?

When given a simple verbal command, such as *tell me your name*, or *blink your eyes*, how does he respond? Consider your patient:
• *alert*, if he responds appropriately to auditory, tactile, and visual stimuli, and is oriented to person, place, and time.
• *lethargic*, if he sleeps a lot, arouses easily, and responds appropriately after he is awakened.
• *obtunded*, if (before he responds appropriately) he needs to be aroused by shaking him or shouting his name. After responding, he'll return to sleep.

If a patient doesn't arouse easily, or responds inappropriately, you'll need to evaluate his response to painful stimuli. For example, when light pressure's applied to his fingernail bed, how does he respond? Consider your patient:
• *stuporous*, if he withdraws his finger or attempts to push your hand away. In most cases, he's never completely awake during stimulation.
• *semicomatose*, if he performs a reflex movement, such as decorticate (flexing one or both arms to his chest), or decerebrate (stiffly extending one or both arms with palms facing outward) posturing.
• *comatose*, if he has no response, no reflexes, and flaccid muscle tone in his extremities.

Be sure to document your patient's level of consciousnness in your nurses' notes. Also include the date and time, your observations, and the stimulus used.

Assessment

Nurses' guide to consciousness grading

Because no universally accepted consciousness grading system exists, use this chart as a guide when assessing your patient's consciousness level.

Remember: If your patient has paralysis or aphasia, you'll need to consider these factors in your final evaluation.

● ● ● Responds normally
● ● Responds with stimulation
● Responds with maximal stimulation
— Does not respond

	Environmental awareness	Speaking ability	Response to spoken word	Pain response	Motor response
Alert	● ● ●	● ● ●	● ● ●	● ● ●	● ● ●
Lethargic	●	● ●	● ●	● ● ●	● ● ●
Obtunded	●	● ●	●	● ●	● ●
Stuporous	—	—	●	● ●	● ●
Semicomatose	—	—	—	●	●
Comatose	—	—	—	—	—

Preparing for neurologic assessment

Up to this point, you've based the initial assessment on data collected from observing, interviewing, and examining your patient. But now you're ready to expand your data baseline by identifying your patient's specific problems. To do this, you'll thoroughly assess his cranial nerves, cerebellar function, motor function, and his sensory function.

Then, regardless of your findings, clearly and thoroughly document all data collected including your observations, the results of your interview, history taking, and general, emotional, cranial nerve, and motor function assessment.

Assessing your patient's olfactory nerve

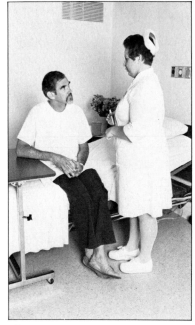

1 *You'll want to begin Mr. Boyle's cranial nerve assessment with the olfactory or first cranial nerve, which controls his sense of smell. Here's how to proceed:*

First, obtain three substances with distinctive, but familiar, odors; for example, coffee, tobacco, and cloves.

▤ *Nursing tip:* If these substances are not readily available, use items in your patient's room, such as flowers, a bar of soap, and mouthwash.

Explain the procedure to Mr. Boyle and have him sit at the edge of the bed, or on a chair. Make sure he's comfortable.

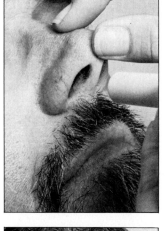

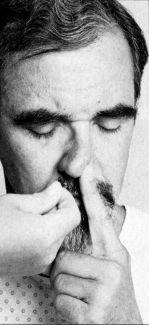

2 Then, examine both his nostrils with a penlight to be certain they're not obstructed. In addition, ask him to alternately occlude each nostril and inhale through the other.

3 Now, ask Mr. Boyle to close his eyes and occlude his left nostril with his finger. Then, hold one of the substances under his right nostril and ask him to identify the odor. To avoid having him inhale the substance, place it near—but not right under—his nostril. Follow this procedure with the other two substances.

Repeat the entire test on his left nostril. Document all test results in your nurses' notes.

Suppose your patient's unable to identify one or more test substances correctly. He may have an olfactory nerve impairment. While a temporal lobe lesion may cause olfactory hallucinations, other possible causes of olfactory impairment are a common cold; allergies; head trauma resulting in parosmia (perversion of the sense of smell); compression of the olfactory bulb by meningiomas or anterior fossa aneurysm; and tumor infiltration in the frontal lobe.

Assessing your patient's optic nerve

1 *Next, you'll need to assess Mr. Boyle's optic or second cranial nerve. As you know, this sensory nerve helps provide your patient's visual acuity, visual fields, and internal eye structure. So, you'll be performing several tests and evaluating the results independently and together.*

Remember: If your patient's wearing corrective lenses, test his acuity with and without the lenses.

First, make sure your patient's seated comfortably in a well-lighted area. Ask him to cover his left eye, without creating pressure. Then, test his visual acuity using a Snellen chart. If his vision's normal, he'll be able to read the line marked 20/20. If he can't, note the smallest line he can read. Then, test his left eye, using the same procedure.

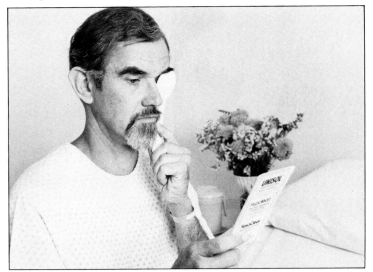

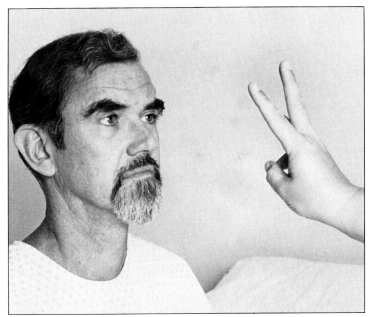

2 Suppose no chart's available. In this case, hold up two fingers and have your patient identify the number of fingers you're holding up. Or, if there is a picture on the wall in his room, ask him to describe it.

3 Now, you're ready to test Mr. Boyle's visual fields. Instruct your patient to cover his right eye with his hand. Take care he's not pressing in on the eye. Close your left eye. Position yourself at eye level with your patient, and approximately 24″ (61 cm) away. Then, ask your patient to look directly into your open eye.

Hold a test object, such as a pencil or finger, at arm's length above your head.

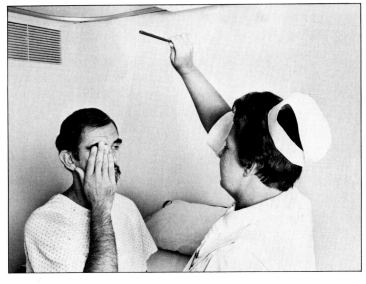

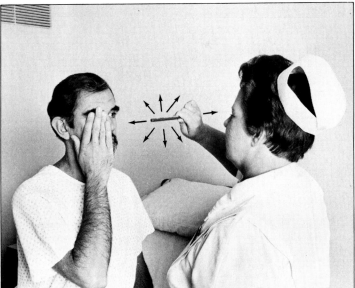

4 Next, lower the pencil from the periphery into your patient's field of vision. Ask him to indicate when he first sees the pencil. Compare this point to the point where *you* first see the pencil, and note any differences.

Repeat this test for each direction shown by these arrows.

Note: When testing your patient's temporal visual field, you'll need to start with the pencil behind him. But, remember, this will bring the pencil into your line of vision first.

When you've completed testing your patient's left eye, repeat the entire examination on his right eye, with his left eye covered. Document your findings.

Assessment

Assessing your patient's optic nerve continued

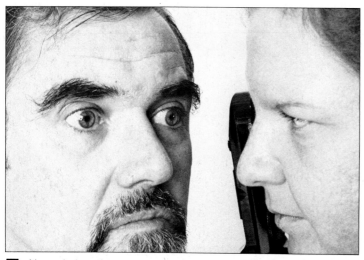

5 Now, darken the room and use an ophthalmoscope to examine your patient's internal eye structure. (For details on using an ophthalmoscope, see the NURSING PHOTOBOOK ASSESSING YOUR PATIENT.) Any abnormalities may be of neurologic origin.

Important: Never use mydriatic drugs to dilate your patient's pupils. This drug may hide changes in his pupils and retinal field.

During the examination, you'll be evaluating your patient's fundus (retina and disc). Expect the retina to be transparent, although pigmentation may vary with race and complexion. The optic disc, which lies where the optic nerve meets the retina, should appear yellowish, and round or oval-shaped. Suppose the disc appears elevated, and pink or engorged with blood (hyperemic) from retinal vessels. Suspect papilledema or choked disc, which is a swelling of the optic nerve tissues caused by increased intracranial pressure.

Expect to see tiny blood vessels surrounding the optic nerve. If no vessels are present—and the optic disc appears white—your patient may have optic atrophy.

Finally, look at the physiologic cup, or depression, which is the small yellowish-white area inside the optic disc. The cup's usually less than half the size of the disc. If the physiologic cup appears unusually small, the optic disc's hyperemic, and your patient has vision loss, he may have papillitis.

Remember to document all findings from your tests in your notes.

Evaluating possible visual field disturbances

If your patient has difficulty performing visual field tests, he may have a visual field disorder. Review the questions below to determine possible causes of these disorders:

• Does your patient have a blind spot in the affected eye? If so, he may have a retinal lesion.
• Does your patient have partial or complete blindness in that eye? If so, he may have an optic nerve lesion.
• Does your patient have blindness in the opposite half of

both visual fields? If so, he may have a lesion of one optic tract or one lateral geniculate body.
• Does your patient have contralateral blindness in the corresponding lower quadrants of his eyes? If so, he may have a parietal lobe lesion.
• Does your patient have contralateral blindness in the corresponding half of each visual field, but not in his central vision? If so, he may have an occipital lobe lesion.

Assessing your patient's oculomotor, trochlear, and abducens nerves

1 *This photostory will show you how to assess Mr. Boyle's oculomotor, trochlear, and abducens nerves. These nerves, also known as the third, fourth, and sixth cranial nerves, help innervate the muscles needed for eye movements. In addition, the oculomotor nerve also innervates the muscles which help regulate pupil constriction and eyelid movement.*

Remember: Because these nerves operate as a unit, you'll test and evaluate them together.

Begin by familiarizing yourself with the six cardinal fields of gaze, shown in this photo. Keep in mind that each of these fields corresponds to one of Mr. Boyle's extraocular muscles. So, you'll want to check each field of gaze separately.

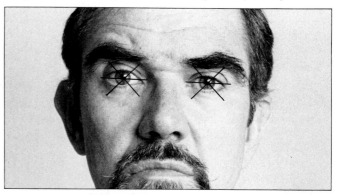

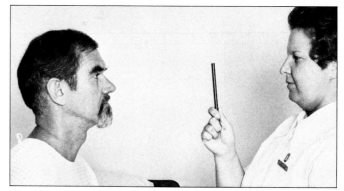

2 Hold a pencil or your finger about 12" (30 cm) in front of your patient's nose.

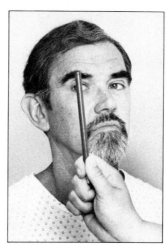

3 Now, ask Mr. Boyle to hold his head still and follow the pencil's movement with his eyes. As you slowly move the pencil to his right, watch his eyes simultaneously.

When the pencil's about 24" (61 cm) from the starting point—or the movement in either of Mr. Boyle's eyes stops—hold the pencil still. Note the position of your patient's iris in relation to each eye's midline.

Repeat this procedure for each of the remaining cardinal fields of gaze.

4 To evaluate your results, imagine your patient's eyeball as a grid divided into quarters, as shown here. If his extraocular movements are within normal ranges, the edge of his iris will approach the grid's center as he moves his eyes.

But, if you see eye jerking, oscillation, sluggish eyelid movement, or if your patient's eyes are not tracking together, suspect possible extraocular muscle problems.

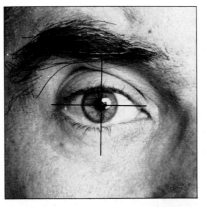

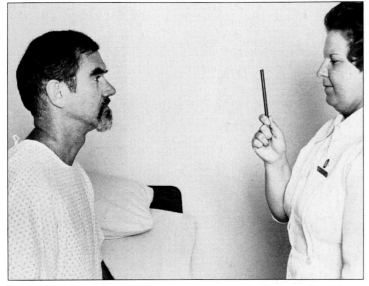

5 Now you're ready to assess Mr. Boyle's extrinsic eye muscles. To do this, hold the pencil about 18″ (46 cm) in front of his nose and note his ability to focus on the pencil.

6 Keeping the pencil in place, test his accommodation and convergence. Ask your patient to keep his head still and follow the pencil with his eyes as you move it.

Then, move the pencil toward the bridge of your patient's nose, as shown here. Both your patient's eyes should converge on the pencil at the same level and distance. When they do, expect his pupils to constrict and remain constricted.

If everything's okay, your patient will be able to sustain his gaze when the pencil is 2″ to 3″ (5.1 to 7.6 cm) from the bridge of his nose.

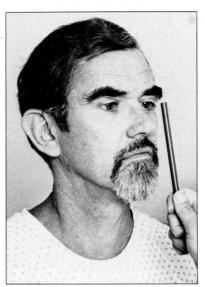

7 Next you'll need to test Mr. Boyle's pupillary light responses which include *direct* and *consensual* reflexes. To begin, note each pupil's size and shape, and their equality. (For details on measuring pupil size, see page 22.) Then, darken the room.

To test your patient's direct light reflex, instruct him to cover his left eye with his hand. Hold his right eyelid open with your hand.

Then, holding the penlight at an angle, direct the light into his right pupil, as shown here. His pupil should constrict quickly and remain so until the light's removed. To minimize your patient's discomfort, avoid shining the light into his eye longer than necessary.

Repeat the procedure on your patient's left pupil with his right eye covered.

Important: If your patient has a glass eye, cataracts, or contact lenses, his pupillary response may be altered or absent.

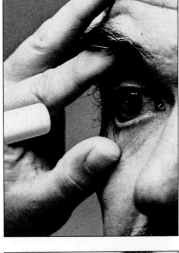

8 Now, to assess Mr. Boyle's consensual light reflex, keep the room darkened. Instruct him to keep both eyes open.

Angle the penlight in front of his right eye as described above. Then, turn on the penlight and note the reaction of the *left* pupil. Expect both pupils to constrict bilaterally until you remove the light.

Then, check his right pupillary response by placing the penlight in front of his other eye. Now, document your findings in your nurses' notes. Also, be sure to ask Mr. Boyle if he experienced any diplopia (double vision) as you performed these tests. If he did, ask him to describe it. Remember, diplopia may indicate oculomotor, trochlear, or abducens nerve damage.

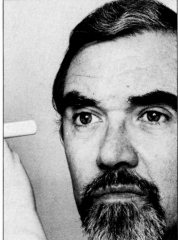

If, during any of these tests, you observe either of Mr. Boyle's eyes deviating inward toward his nose, suspect abducens nerve damage. Was Mr. Boyle unable to move either eye down or laterally? If so, suspect trochlear nerve damage. And, if you note ptosis; a dilated pupil unreactive to light; nystagmus; or an inability to move either eye medially, or up or down normally; it may indicate oculomotor nerve damage.

But remember, always ask your patient if he's taking any medication. While nystagmus may be from a posterior fossa lesion, it can also be from drug toxicity: for example, caused by an anticonvulsant, such as phenytoin sodium (Dilantin*).

Finally, some additional causes of oculomotor, trochlear, and abducens nerve damage may be: trauma, multiple sclerosis, tumor or aneurysm at the base of the skull, botulism, or lead poisoning.

*Available in both the United States and in Canada

Assessment

A closer look at the pupils

Up to now you've assessed your patient's visual acuity, visual fields, and internal eye structure. But now you'll want to accurately measure your patient's pupil size. Why? To use as a baseline for your ongoing patient assessment. As you know, a change in your patient's pupil size may indicate a change in his neurologic condition.

When documenting pupil size, avoid using vague terms, such as constricted or dilated. These words may mean different things to different nurses. Instead, document your patient's exact pupil size, using the chart below as a guide.

But remember, normal pupil sizes range from 1.5 mm to 6 mm, and vary from patient to patient. So, try to establish what's normal for your patient and document your measurements carefully. For more information on pupillary abnormalities, see the neurocheck (neurowatch) section of this book.

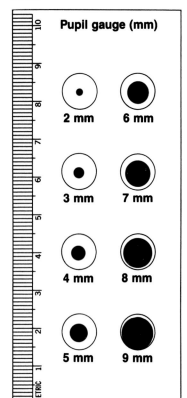

Pupil gauge (mm)

2 mm   6 mm

3 mm   7 mm

4 mm   8 mm

5 mm   9 mm

Assessing your patient's trigeminal nerve

1 *To properly assess Mr. Boyle's facial sensitivity, you must test his trigeminal, or fifth cranial nerve. To do this, you'll need to evaluate his reaction to various types of sensation. As you do, always note whether both sides of his face are equally sensitive. Proceed as follows:*

Begin by gathering this equipment: two test tubes or small bottles, safety pin, and reflex hammer. You'll also need a cotton ball. Instruct your patient to close his eyes and keep them closed until you tell him to open them.

Important: If your patient has suspected trigeminal neuralgia, be very careful when testing facial sensitivity. Temperature differences, and the pin's sharpness may aggravate any pain he's experiencing.

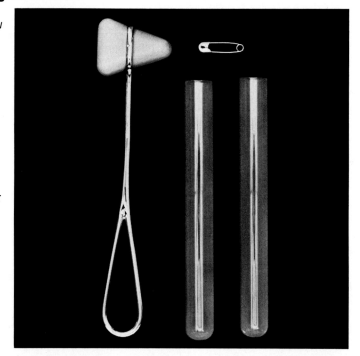

2 Now, use a cotton wisp to touch first one side of his forehead, and then the other. Ask your patient to tell you when and where he feels the cotton.

Repeat the test on his cheeks and jaw.

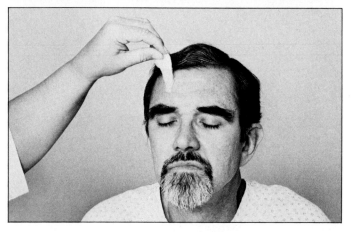

3 To test Mr. Boyle's temperature sensitivity, fill one test tube with hot water and the other with cold water.

First, touch the test tube filled with hot water to one side of Mr. Boyle's face. Hold it there for about 1 second.

Touch the test tube filled with cold water to the same area and hold it there for 1 second. Repeat the procedure on the opposite side of Mr. Boyle's face. Ask him to tell you what he feels, and where he feels it. If his sensory perception's normal, he'll be able to distinguish between hot and cold.

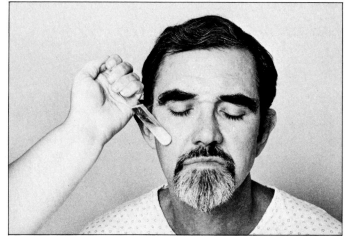

4 Next, assess Mr. Boyle's facial sensation by gently touching one side of his forehead with the sharp end of a safety pin. As you do, ask him to tell you what he feels, and where he feels it. He should experience pain if everything's okay.

Touch the same side of his forehead with the pin's dull end. Ask your patient to describe what he's feeling, including whether the sensation is sharp or dull. If his sensory perception's normal, he'll be able to distinguish between sharp and dull sensations equally on both sides.

Repeat the test on both sides of your patient's cheeks and jaw, and compare your findings.

Instruct your patient to open his eyes.

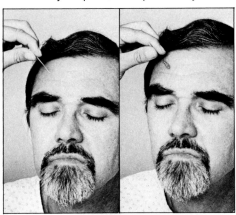

5 Now you're ready to assess Mr. Boyle's corneal reflex. To do this, ask him to look up. Approaching from his right side, gently touch his right cornea—but not the conjunctiva—with a cotton wisp. Be careful not to touch his eyelashes or his sclera. Your patient's eye should blink and tear when the cornea's touched.

Important: If your patient wears contact lenses, his corneal reflexes may be diminished or totally absent.

Repeat the test on his left cornea.

6 Next, instruct Mr. Boyle to clench his teeth. The ability to clench your teeth indicates an intact motor function.

Then, palpate his temporal muscles on his right and left temples, as shown here. Both muscles should feel equal in size and strength.

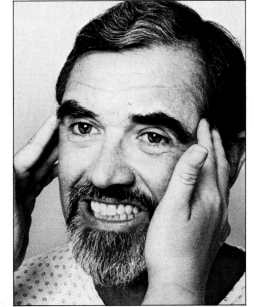

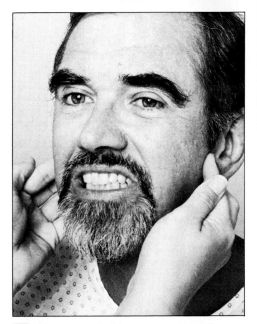

7 Now, palpate his masseter muscles, located on either side of his jaw joints. These muscles should also be equal in size and strength.

Note: If your patient wears dentures or has no teeth, his motor function assessment may be decreased.

8 Now, as he continues to clench his teeth, test your patient's pterygoid muscle strength. Grasp his lower jaw with one hand and pull downward. If everything's okay, your patient will be able to keep his teeth clenched, resisting your efforts.

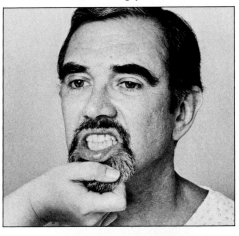

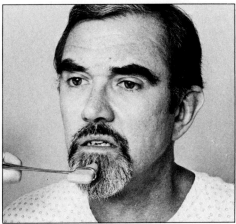

9 Next, tell your patient to unclench his teeth and open his mouth slightly. Assess his maxillary reflex, or jaw jerk, by tapping the middle of his chin with a reflex hammer. You should see a sudden, slight closing of his jaw.

Remember to document all test results in your notes.

Absence of any of these test responses may indicate a trigeminal nerve tumor. For example, a lesion of the pons produces masticatory muscle paralysis and light-touch sensation loss in the face, while a medulla lesion affecting the descending tract causes pain and produces a loss of temperature sensation and corneal reflex.

As you probably know, trigeminal nerve damage can be caused by trauma, trigeminal neuralgia (tic douloureux), a meningeal infection, an intracranial aneurysm, or multiple sclerosis.

Assessment

Assessing your patient's facial nerves

1 *Do you know how to assess Mr. Boyle's facial expressions and sense of taste? As you know, these functions are provided by the facial or seventh cranial nerve. If you're unsure, read this story to learn how.*

First, observe your patient's face while at rest and as he talks. Then, ask him to raise his eyebrows, frown, smile, and puff out his cheeks. Note any asymmetry or abnormal movements.

Now you're ready to test the upper motor portion of Mr. Boyle's facial nerve. Ask your patient to close his eyes tightly. Tell him to keep them closed while you try to open them, as shown.

2 Next, test the lower portion of your patient's facial nerve by having Mr. Boyle puff out his cheeks. Instruct him to resist your efforts to collapse them, as shown here. If you notice facial asymmetry, abnormal movements (such as tics), or both during this part of the assessment, suspect a facial nerve lesion.

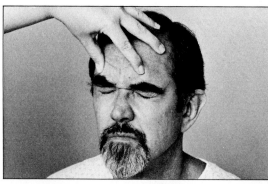

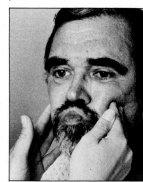

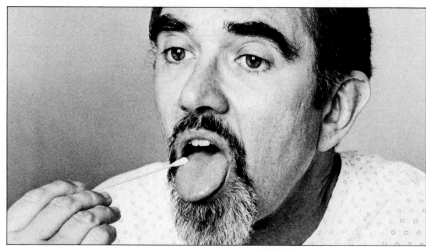

3 Check the sensory portion of your patient's facial nerve. Do this by dipping a cotton swab into sugar. Then, ask your patient to stick out his tongue. Touch the swab to one side of the anterior part of his tongue on each side. Tell him to keep his tongue out until he tastes the flavor. If he pulls in his tongue or swallows prematurely, the test substance may spread to the opposite side of his tongue, giving false test results of your patient's tasting ability.

Now, ask him to identify the flavor. *Note:* If your patient's sense of smell is impaired, he may lose his ability to taste. Then, instruct him to rinse his mouth with water. Repeat the procedure, substituting salt.

In many cases, an inability to correctly identify both flavors indicates a lesion in the facial nerve sensory fibers or sensory nucleus. Facial nerve injury may result from trauma to peripheral nerve branches, mastoid surgery complications, temporal bone fracture, intracerebral bleeds, parotid area lacerations, or contusions. Other possible causes of facial nerve abnormalities may include intracranial tumor, meningitis, herpes zoster, or Bell's palsy.

Document all results in your notes.

Assessing your patient's acoustic nerve: the preliminaries

1 *Ready to assess Mr. Boyle's hearing and equilibrium? Begin by examining his ear canals with an otoscope to rule out any physical abnormalities which may affect his hearing or equilibrium.*

As you look through the otoscope, expect to see brown or orange wax (cerumen) along the smooth, pink walls. Remember, excessive wax accumulation or blockage may alter your patient's equilibrium or affect his hearing.

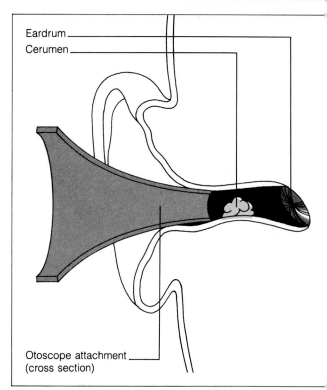

Eardrum

Cerumen

Otoscope attachment
(cross section)

2 Expect Mr. Boyle's eardrum to appear as a pearl gray or pale pink disc that's slightly coned inward. Behind the eardrum you'll see the malleus handle which points downward in the center of your patient's eardrum.

If the eardrum's properly positioned, look for a

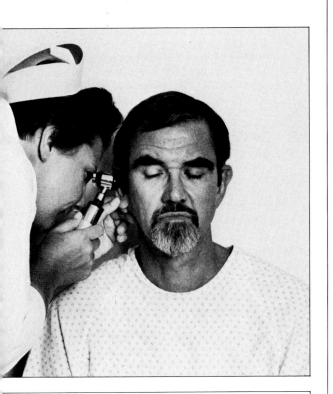

Malleus

Incus

Malleus handle

Cone of light

cone of light at the 5 o'clock position in the right ear (as shown), and at the 7 o'clock position in the left ear. If the cone of light is displaced or absent, his eardrum may be bulging, retracted, or inflamed. Any of these conditions may affect his hearing or balance. Document your findings.

Assessing your patient's acoustic nerve: testing hearing and equilibrium

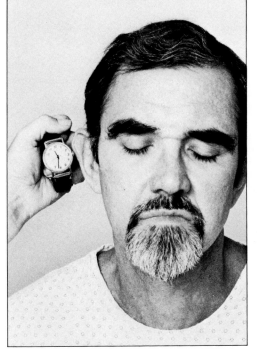

1 *Now you're ready to test your patient's acoustic or eighth cranial nerve. The acoustic nerve actually consists of the cochlear nerve, which provides hearing ability, and the vestibular nerve, which controls equilibrium. Because the vestibular nerve is not tested routinely, we'll just show you how to test the cochlear nerve in this photostory. Follow these steps:*
To determine Mr. Boyle's normal hearing ability, place a ticking watch close to his right ear.

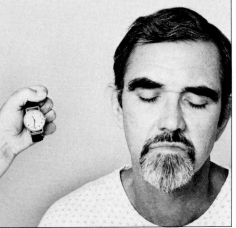

2 If your patient can hear the ticking, gradually move the watch away from his ear. Ask him to tell you when he can no longer hear the ticking. He should hear the ticking a maximum of 4″ to 6″ (10.2 to 15.2 cm) from his ear. Repeat the test on his left ear.
Note: You may also perform the hearing test by holding the watch away from his ear, moving it toward his ear, and asking him to tell you when he first hears the ticking.

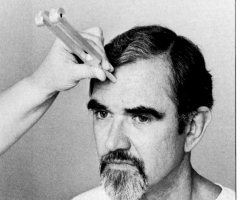

3 To test for lateralization (Weber test), place the base of a vibrating tuning fork on top of your patient's forehead, as shown here. Ask Mr. Boyle if the tone is centralized or referred to the left or right side. He should hear the same tone (volume and intensity) in each ear. If he does, document the result as Weber negative.
But, if he hears the tone louder in one ear, ask him which ear has the louder tone. Then, document this result as Weber right or Weber left.

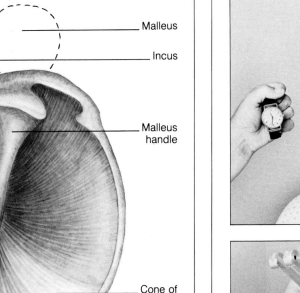

Assessment

Assessing your patient's acoustic nerve: testing hearing and equilibrium continued

4 Now you're ready to perform the Rinne test. As you know, this test compares the strength of Mr. Boyle's hearing through bone conduction to that of air conduction.

To test bone conduction, touch the base of the vibrating tuning fork to your patient's right mastoid process. If all's well, he'll hear the tone immediately. Ask him to tell you when he no longer hears the tone, and note this amount of time.

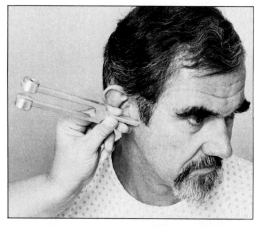

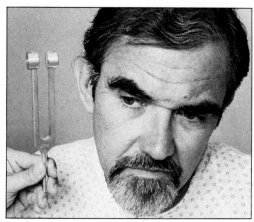

5 Then, without vibrating the fork again, assess air conduction by holding the vibrating prongs ½″ (1.3 cm) next to your patient's right external ear canal. Make sure the prongs are in front of, but not touching, the ear canal.

Ask him to tell you when he no longer hears the tone. Also, note this length of time. Normally, your patient will hear the tone carried by air conduction twice as long as the tone carried by bone conduction.

Repeat the procedure on his left ear.

Document all results in your nurses' notes. Although tinnitus, decreased hearing, or deafness may indicate cochlear nerve damage, other possible causes of abnormal test findings include inflammation, intracranial tumor, drug toxicity, and middle fossa skull fracture.

Assessing your patient's glossopharyngeal and vagus nerves

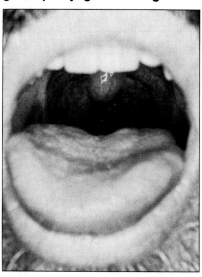

1 *Now we'll show you how to assess your patient's glossopharyngeal and vagus, or ninth and tenth cranial nerves. These nerves help regulate Mr. Boyle's gag and palatal reflexes and work as a unit. So, you'll always test these nerves together. Here's how to proceed:*

To assess the vagus nerve, ask Mr. Boyle to yawn or say "ah." As he does, observe his soft palate and uvula for upward movement, and his posterior pharynx for inward movement. Note any asymmetry.

Then, ask your patient to speak and swallow. His voice should be clear and without hoarseness.

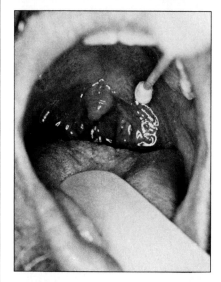

2 Now, assess Mr. Boyle's gag reflex. To do this, ask him to open his mouth. Then, hold down his tongue with a tongue depressor. Use a cotton swab to touch each side of his pharynx. His gag reflex should be immediate. *Note:* If your patient's elderly, expect a weakened gag reflex.

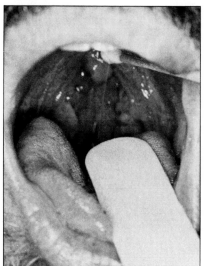

3 To assess your patient's palatal reflex, instruct him to open his mouth again. Touch each side of the uvula with a cotton swab. The uvula should rise.

Was Mr. Boyle's voice hoarse or nasal sounding? If so, suspect nerve damage. He may have ninth or tenth cranial nerve damage if pharyngeal stimulation leads to impaired gagging and increased mucus in his mouth; or if his soft palate is immobile. What causes ninth cranial nerve damage? Acute anterior poliomyelitis, intramedullary lesions, syringobulbia, vascular lesions, and multiple sclerosis may cause impaired test responses. Infection or intracranial tumors may cause tenth cranial nerve damage.

Document everything in your nurses' notes.

Assessing your patient's spinal accessory nerve

1 *Now you'll need to assess Mr. Boyle's spinal accessory, or 11th cranial nerve. To do this, you'll test his trapezius and sternocleidomastoid muscles which allow his head to rotate and nod. Here's how:*

Begin by testing the strength of your patient's trapezius muscle. Stand facing your patient and place your hands on Mr. Boyle's shoulders, as shown here.

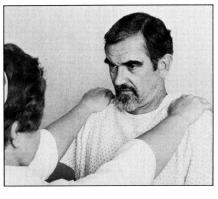

2 Then, instruct him to raise his shoulders as you apply downward pressure.

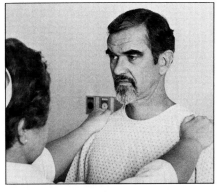

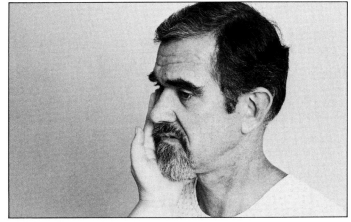

3 To test Mr. Boyle's sternocleidomastoid muscle strength, remain standing and place your left hand on the right side of your patient's face. Tell him to turn his head against your hand's pressure. Then, repeat the procedure on the left side of his face.

If either the trapezius or sternocleidomastoid muscle seems abnormally weak, or if a muscle on one side seems longer than one on the other side, suspect a lesion. Other possible causes of abnormalities include: occipital bone necrosis, inflammation, syringobulbia, amyotrophic lateral sclerosis, and demyelinating diseases of the medulla.

Document the findings in your notes.

Assessing your patient's hypoglossal nerve

1 *To accurately assess your patient's hypoglossal (12th cranial) nerve, you must test his tongue's movement and strength. Follow these steps.*

To begin, ask your patient to open his mouth. Examine his tongue as it lies on the floor of his mouth. It should lie flat with no tremors or twitching.

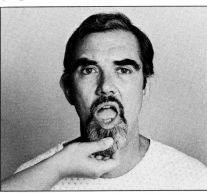

2 Now, ask your patient to stick out his tongue. It should protrude centered between his lips. Note any tremor or atrophy.

Next, tell your patient to quickly dart his tongue in and out of his mouth. Then, have him stick out his tongue and move it from side to side as quickly as he can. The tongue movements should be smooth and fast.

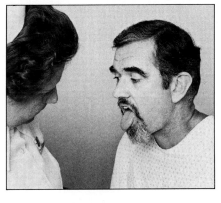

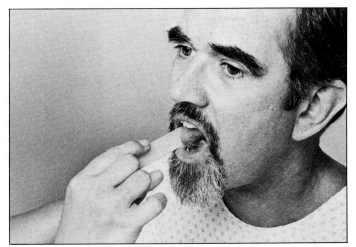

3 To test your patient's tongue strength, you'll need a tongue depressor. Hold the depressor on one side of his mouth and ask him to push against it with his tongue. Then, repeat the procedure on the other side of his mouth.

Is your patient unable to move his tongue toward one side of his mouth or the other? Or, do you note fasciculations, tremors, or an increased wrinkling of the tongue's surface? If so, suspect a nerve lesion. Other possible causes of these abnormalities include: syringobulbia, amyotrophic lateral sclerosis, alcoholism, or cerebrovascular accident.

Remember to document all results in your notes.

Assessment

Assessing your patient's cerebellar function

1 *Now that you've completed Mr. Boyle's cranial nerve testing, you're ready to assess his cerebellar function and nerve pathway integrity. As you know, the cerebellum controls coordination and balance. While testing your patient, keep in mind how accurately and* smoothly he performs each action. Proceed as follows:

Begin by testing Mr. Boyle's hand-eye coordination. Ask him to touch his nose, first with his right hand, then his left hand. Have him repeat the test with his eyes closed.

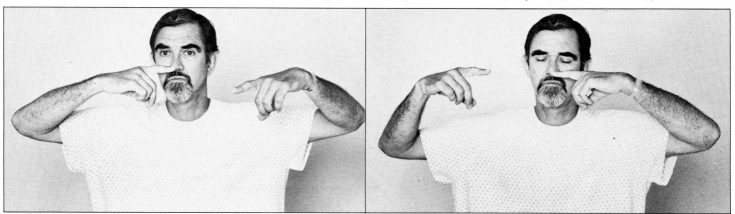

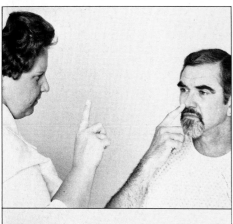

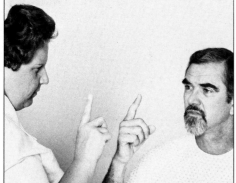

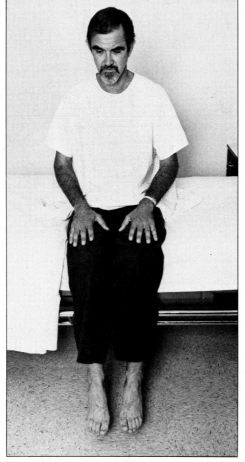

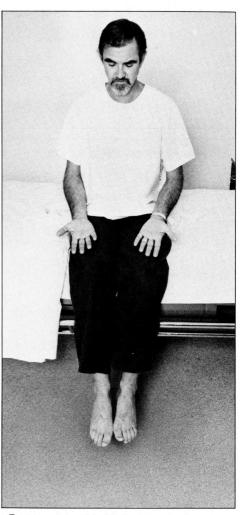

2 Now, place your finger about 18″ (46 cm) in front of your patient's face (top photo). Instruct him to repeatedly touch first the tip of his nose—then your fingertip—with his right hand (bottom photo). As he does, change your finger's position. Note his ability to gauge distance, as well as any tremor, or difficulty he has with the procedure.

Repeat the test with his left hand.

3 Next, test Mr. Boyle's arm and hand coordination by performing the following three tests. First, ask him to quickly and repeatedly pat both his thighs with his hands. Note any slowness, difficulty, or lack of coordination.

4 Now, have Mr. Boyle repeatedly pat both thighs, alternating his palms up and then down, as quickly as he can.

5 For the third test, tell your patient to sequentially touch his thumbs to each of the four fingers on the corresponding hand, as quickly as possible.

Be sure to note and document any slowness or other difficulties.

Keep in mind during all three tests that Mr. Boyle's dominant hand may perform better than his nondominant hand.

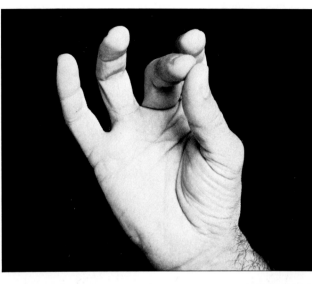

6 Now, instruct your patient to place his right heel on his left knee, as shown here. Tell him to slide his heel down his shin. Document any problems. Have him repeat the test with his left foot.

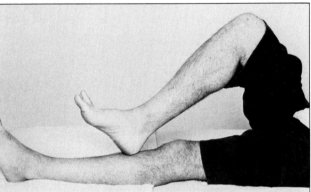

7 Ask Mr. Boyle to form an imaginary figure eight in the air with his right foot. Tell him to continue to do so for about 30 seconds. Then, have him repeat the same test with his left foot . Does he have any difficulty? If so, note it.

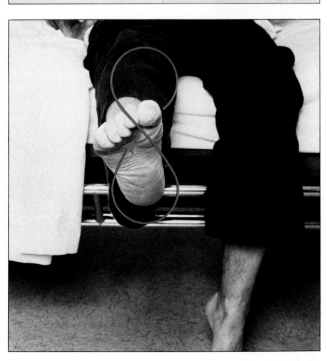

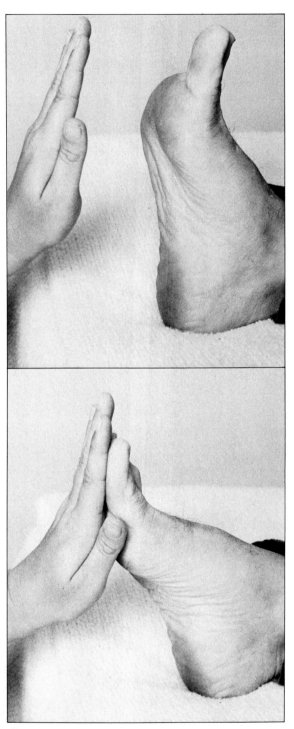

8 Now, have your patient lie down on the bed. Place a pillow under his head.

Standing at the end of the bed, put your left hand about 4″ (10.2 cm) from the ball of his right foot (see top photo). Ask him to touch your hand with the ball of his foot (bottom photo). Note if he has difficulty following your instructions.

Repeat the test on his left foot.

Assessment

9 Next, you'll need to perform the Romberg test. To do this, ask Mr. Boyle to stand with his feet together and his arms at his sides. His eyes should be open. Carefully note his posture and balance.

Note: If your patient's wearing shoes, have him remove them. Doing so allows you to more accurately assess neurologic disorders.

Now, ask your patient to close his eyes and remain standing, as shown. Compare his balance with his eyes closed to that with his eyes open. Expect to see slight side-to-side swaying.

Important: Remain close to Mr. Boyle to prevent injury from a loss of balance.

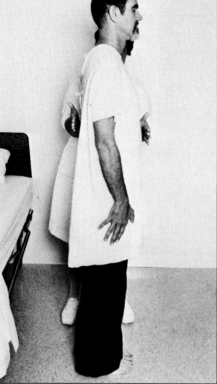

10 Suppose you observe excessive swaying (Romberg's sign). You'll want to further assess his balance, by asking him to hop on his right foot (if he's physically able). Then, have him hop on his left foot. He should be able to maintain his balance on each foot.

Note: An inability to hop or maintain balance while hopping may also result from arthritis or old age.

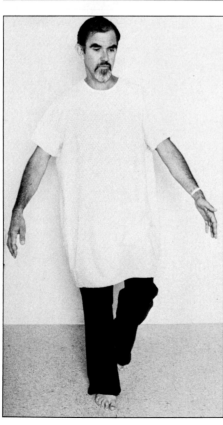

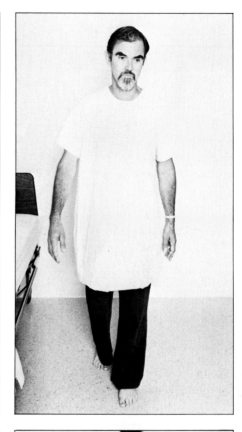

11 Now, with your patient's eyes open, have him walk across the room. As he does, note his gait, balance, arm swing, and posture.

Then, have him walk with his eyes closed. Again, compare the two results.

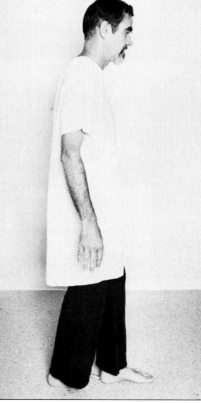

12 Finally, instruct your patient to walk in tandem fashion (heel-to-toe) across the room. As before, observe his posture, balance, and arm swing. You should see some side-to-side swaying.

Remember to document all results in your nurses' notes. If, during any of these tests, Mr. Boyle has tremors, ataxia, or difficulty with alternating movement (such as pronation and supination), it may indicate cerebellar involvement. All three symptoms are common to cerebellar disease. Other symptoms may include nystagmus, and speech and muscle tone abnormalities.

Assessing your patient's motor system

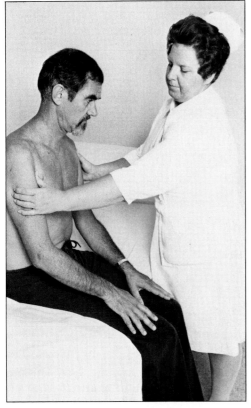

1 *When you assessed Mr. Boyle's cerebellar function, you examined his nervous system above the spinal cord. Now, we'll show you how to assess Mr. Boyle's motor system. Along with the sensory system, it composes the nervous system below the spinal cord.*

To assess your patient's motor system, you'll need to evaluate muscle size, involuntary movement, tone, and strength. Here's how:

First, instruct your patient to sit at the edge of his bed or on a chair with his arms at his sides. Note symmetry of posture, muscle contour, and outline.

Then, inspect and palpate his muscles for size, consistency, and atrophy. Be sure to note your findings. Do you see any abnormal voluntary or involuntary movements such as rapid and continuous twitching, tremors, tics, or rapid and jerky movements? If so, these abnormalities may indicate a disturbance of the extrapyramidal motor areas or their pathways.

Note: Tics and other abnormal involuntary movements may be caused by emotional problems.

Examine the fine muscles of your patient's hand. Note any wasting, fasciculations, or fine tremors. But remember, fasciculations with muscle wasting may appear in lower motor neuron disorders.

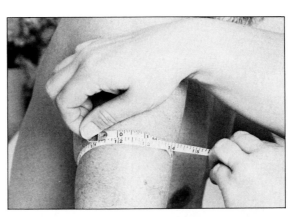

2 Next, use a tape measure to measure the muscle in Mr. Boyle's upper right arm. Then, measure the muscle at the same location in his other arm. Compare both measurements and note any differences. Follow this procedure to measure the upper part of his thighs and calves.

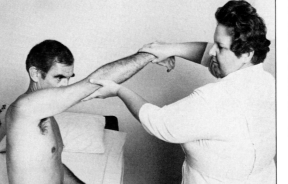

3 Now, have your patient relax. Support his right elbow with one hand, as shown here. Use your other hand to grasp his wrist and bring his arm through a complete range of motion. Note any abnormalities, such as flaccidity, pain, rigidity, jerking, spasticity, and resistance.

Repeat this procedure with his left arm.

4 Next, support your patient's knee with one hand and place your other hand under his heel. Bring his leg through a complete range of motion, again noting any flaccidity, pain, rigidity, jerking, spasticity, or resistance.

Repeat this test on your patient's other leg.

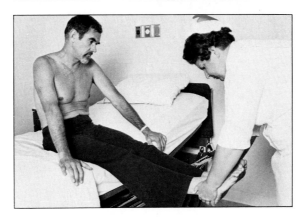

5 If you observe abnormal movement in your patient's arms or legs, perform these tests:

First, have Mr. Boyle sit with his legs dangling over the edge of the bed. Hold his heels with the palms of your hands and lift his heels to knee level.

Remove your hands from his heels and observe his leg movement. His legs should drop freely. If your patient's legs drop only slightly or not at all, note and document the degree of limitation or rigidity.

Assessment

Assessing your patient's motor system continued

6 To test your patient's wrist flexibility, ask him to keep his right arm relaxed. Grasp his arm slightly above his wrist and shake his arm several times. Note the wrist movement. If everything's okay, his wrist will move freely. Note any abnormalities you observe.

Repeat this test on his left wrist.

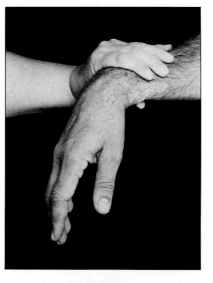

7 Ask your patient to lie flat on the bed. Place one hand under his right knee and the palm of your other hand under his right heel. Lift his foot 12″ (30 cm) off the bed, as shown here.

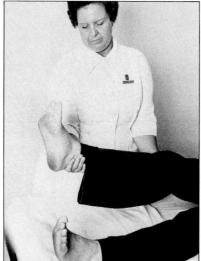

8 Now, keeping your hand under his knee, remove your other hand from his heel. Expect his foot to fall quickly and freely. Does his leg remain extended or fall slowly? If so, he may have rigidity or spasticity.

Repeat the procedure on his left leg.

9 Now you're ready to test your patient's muscle strength.
Note: Never test a patient's muscle strength if you have any muscle weakness yourself. If you do, the muscle strength test results may be inaccurate.

Begin by asking your patient to stand with his eyes closed. Then, have him extend his arms with his palms up, and hold this position for 30 seconds. As he does, note any tendency he has to turn his palms down (pronation), lower his arms, or bend them at the elbows. Also note any tremors or other involuntary movements that may indicate muscle weakness. If muscle weakness is greater in his distal region, it may indicate a neurologic disorder such as myotonic muscular dystrophy (myotonia atrophia).

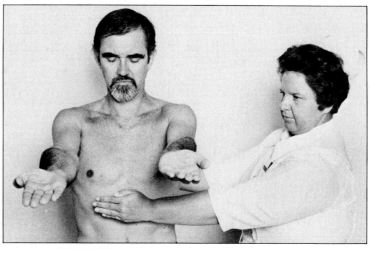

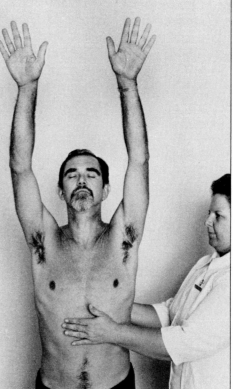

10 Now, ask your patient to keep his eyes closed and extend both his arms above his head with his palms facing forward. Have him maintain this position for 30 seconds. Observe his ability to hold this position, watching for any downward drifting of his arms or hands. If you note weakness on one side, suspect hemiparesis or shoulder-girdle disease.

Now, step behind Mr. Boyle and have him resist your efforts to push his arms to his sides. Note each arm's strength.

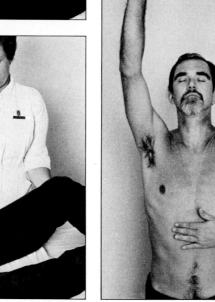

11 Next, have your patient open his eyes and extend his right arm in front of him. Stand behind him, slightly to his right side. Tell him to resist your efforts to push down his extended arm (see photo). Note any weakness. If you observe the tips of Mr. Boyle's shoulder blades protruding abnormally, suspect a serratus anterior muscle weakness.

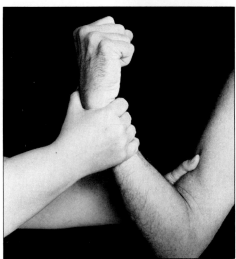

12 Now, test your patient's elbow flexion and extension. To do this, stand at his right side. Hold his upper arm with your left hand and grasp his wrist with your right hand. To test elbow flexion, ask him to pull his arm toward his body as you pull his arm away from his body. Then, have him extend his elbow against your hand's counterpressure.

Repeat the test on his left arm and compare the results.

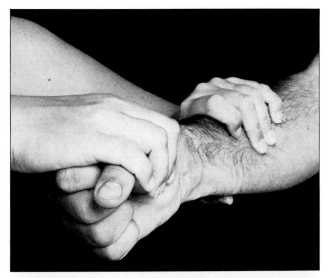

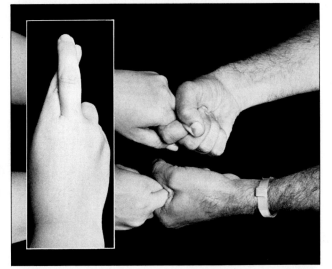

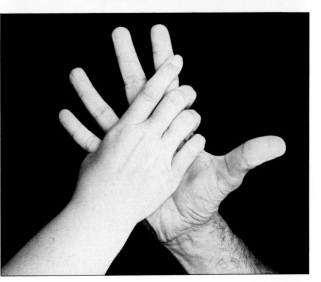

13 To test wrist dorsiflexion, instruct your patient to hold his right arm at his side with his elbow flexed and his forearm extended forward. Ask him to make a fist. Place your left hand on his forearm, just behind his wrist, and your right hand over his fist. Tell him that you'll be pressing down on his hand and want him to resist.

As you exert downward pressure, note your patient's reaction. If Mr. Boyle's wrist is weak, suspect a radial nerve disorder.

Repeat the test on his left arm.

14 Continue the assessment by testing your patient's grip. Hold out your middle and index fingers with the middle finger on top of the index finger (see inset photo). Instruct your patient to grasp your fingers as tightly as he can with his hands. As he does, try pulling your fingers from his grip. You should have difficulty pulling your fingers loose. If his grip is weak, he may have weak forearm muscles or be in pain.

15 Next, to test abduction, ask your patient to spread the fingers of his right hand. Grasp his hand, as shown here. Then, tell him to resist your efforts as you squeeze his fingers as tightly as possible. You should have trouble doing this. If you note any weakness, he may have an ulnar nerve disorder.

Repeat the procedure on his left hand.

Assessment

Assessing your patient's motor system continued

16 Now you're ready to test finger flexion and thumb adduction and opposition. First, ask your patient to press his right thumb against his right fingertips, as shown here. Hook your thumb and index finger through his fingers.

Tell your patient to resist your efforts to separate them. Then, try to pull his thumb and fingers apart. Note any weakness.

Repeat this procedure on his left hand.

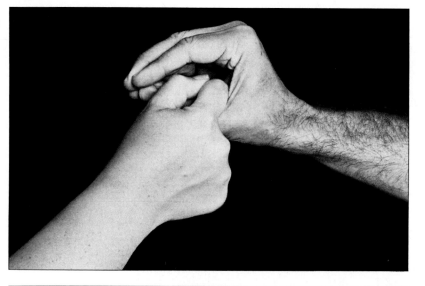

17 To test your patient's hip flexion, ask him to lie flat on his back on the bed. Use one hand to press down on his right thigh as you instruct him to elevate that leg. Note any difficulties he has in doing so.

Repeat the procedure on his left leg.

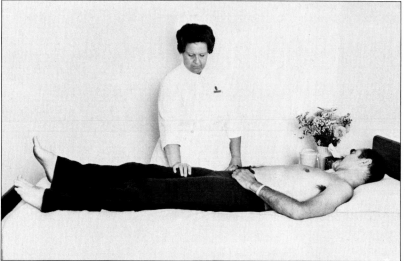

18 Now, test his hip abduction by pressing the outside of his legs together at the knees, as the nurse is doing here. Ask him to try spreading his legs apart, against your pressure. Be sure to note any problems.

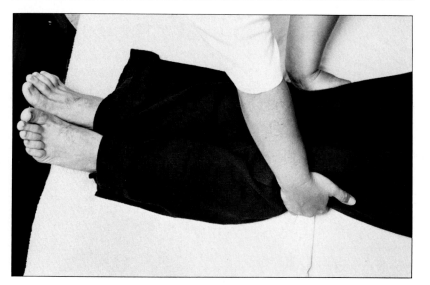

19 Remove your hands and have your patient spread his legs slightly apart. Place your right hand on the inside of his right knee, and your left hand on the inside of his left knee. To assess his hip adduction, ask him to attempt bringing his legs together as you apply outward pressure.

Again, note any difficulties.

20 Now, ask your patient to flex his right leg at the knee and to put his foot flat on the bed. Position your left hand on his raised knee and your right hand over his right Achilles tendon. Then, instruct him to resist your pressure, as you attempt to straighten his leg by pulling his foot outward and pressing down on his knee.

Repeat this test on his left leg.

21 Next, ask your patient to extend both legs flat on the bed. Then, have him raise his right foot off the bed. Put one hand under his right knee and your other hand on his ankle. Tell your patient to resist your efforts to push his foot down on the bed. Then, start applying pressure. Note any problems he has.

Repeat this procedure on his left leg.

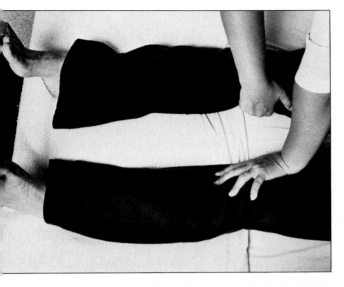

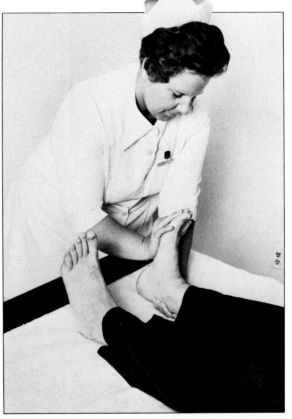

22 Now, with your patient's legs extended flat on the bed, ask him to point his toes upward. Place one hand under his right ankle and the other hand on the ball of his right foot (see photo).

Then, ask your patient to resist your pressure, as you push against his right foot so it flexes toward his knee. Note the results.

Repeat the procedure on his left foot.

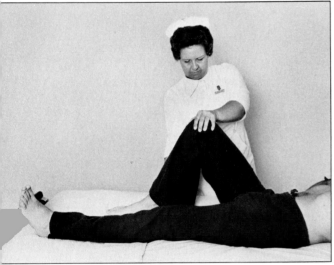

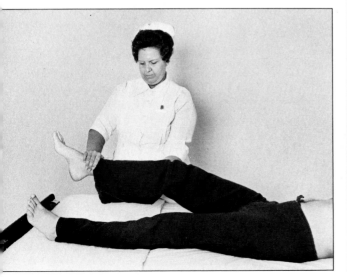

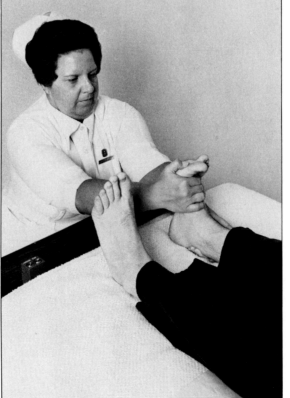

23 Again, position one hand under your patient's right ankle, with your other hand on top of his foot. Then, instruct your patient to resist your effort to flex his foot down.

Repeat the procedure on his left foot.

Finally, document everything in your nurses' notes. Include any evidence of muscle weakness, atrophy, or tremors, which may indicate a lesion in any of the following locations: cerebrum's pyramidal pathway, brain stem, spinal cord, peripheral nerves, neuromuscular junctions, or in the muscle itself.

Assessment

Understanding sensory testing

Your next step in Mr. Boyle's neurologic evaluation is to assess his sensory system. In the story at right, we've divided this sensory system testing into two forms of sensation: primary, and cortical and discriminatory. As you perform each of the sensory system tests, you'll be evaluating your patient for the following factors:
- his ability to perceive and identify each sensation
- his responses on both sides of his body and on his corresponding extremities
- comparable responses for each sensation on the proximal and the distal parts of each extremity
- whether any noted deficiency or disturbance is localized or involves the entire body side.

Assessing your patient's sensory system

1 *To properly perform sensory system assessment, you'll need the following equipment: cotton, applicator stick, key, neurologic pin, forceps, a tuning fork, two test tubes, and three different-sized coins (such as a nickel, dime, and quarter). You'll also need a paper towel or waxed paper to test your patient's texture discrimination. Then, proceed as follows:*

Explain each part of this examination to Mr. Boyle as you perform it. Reassure him that no part of the procedure will hurt him. Then, ask him to close his eyes. Tell your patient that he'll have to keep his eyes closed throughout the sensory testing. In this way, the results will more accurately determine his perception and interpretation of the stimuli.

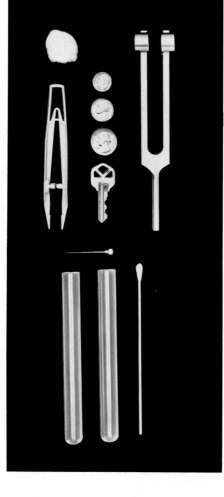

2 Begin your primary sensation assessment by testing Mr. Boyle's tactile sensation. To do this, touch his right hand with a wisp of cotton, as shown here. Ask him to tell you whenever you touch his skin. If your patient doesn't feel any sensation, suspect anesthesia. If he perceives the touch as lighter than it is (less than normal sensation), this indicates hypoesthesia. Suspect hyperesthesia if he perceives the touch as heavier than it is (greater than normal). *Remember:* A decrease in sensation is more common than its total absence. Then, test his left hand as previously described, and compare the results.

Repeat the procedure on your patient's forearms, upper arms, torso, feet, lower legs, and thighs, in that order.

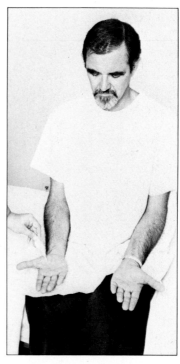

3 Next, test Mr. Boyle's superficial pain sensation. To do this, hold a pin loosely between your fingers. Then, gently touch the point of the pin to his upper right arm. To maintain even pressure, slide your fingers down the pin, and gently press the point against his skin. Continue to do so, occasionally substituting the pin's blunt end. Ask your patient to tell you whether the sensation he feels is sharp or dull.

Note the test results.

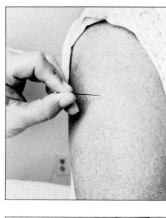

4 To test your patient's temperature sensitivity, you'll need to fill one test tube with hot water and the other with cold water.

Then, ask your patient to lie on the bed. Touch the test tube with hot water to his abdomen, holding it there for about 1 second. Next, touch the cold one to the same location on his abdomen for the same time period. Ask Mr. Boyle to tell you whether he's feeling hot or cold. Be sure to note the results in your notes.

Use the same technique to test other body parts, including his face and extremities.

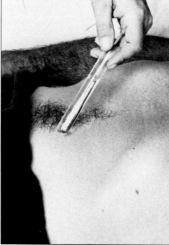

5 Now you're ready to test Mr. Boyle's sensitivity to vibration. To do this, vibrate the tuning fork by tapping it on the heel of your hand. Then, place the base of the fork firmly on the interphalangeal joint of his right great toe, as the nurse is doing here. Ask him to tell you what he's feeling.

To determine if he's feeling pressure or vibration, leave the fork in place and stop the vibration by placing your hand over the fork. Again, ask him what he feels. Then, test his left great toe.

Repeat the tests on the bony prominences of his wrists, shoulders, hips, ankles, shins, knees, and elbows.

6 Next, test your patient's response to deep-pressure pain. Do this by squeezing his Achilles tendon on his right ankle. Ask him to tell you when he feels the pressure. Repeat the test on his left Achilles tendon.

Using the same procedure, test your patient's calf and forearm muscles.

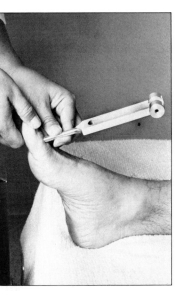

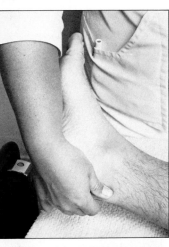

7 To test Mr. Boyle's motion and position sensitivity, hold his right index finger between your thumb and index finger, as shown here. Now, slowly move his finger up, then down. As you do, ask him to tell you whether his finger is being moved up or down.

Suppose your patient has difficulty differentiating directions. In this case, repeat the test by proceeding proximally to his right wrist and elbow. *Note:* Always support the area above the joint being tested.

Repeat the test on his left finger. Then, use the same procedure to test your patient's legs. First, repeat the test on his right and left toes, and if necessary, on his ankles and knees.

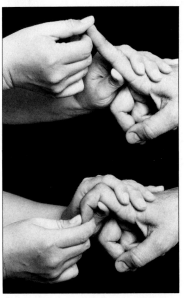

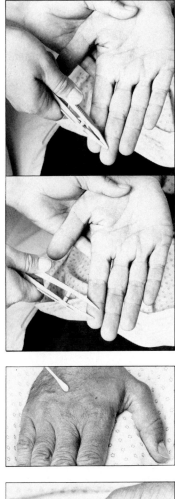

8 Now you'll need to test Mr. Boyle's cortical and discriminatory sensations. Remind your patient to keep his eyes closed. Then, test his two-point discrimination. To do this, simultaneously touch two points on his fingers with the forceps, as shown here.

Then, touch just one spot on his finger. He should be able to differentiate one touch from the two simultaneous touches. Ask him to tell you whether he feels one or two touches.

Next, repeat the test, changing the distance between the two touches. If everything's okay, your patient will distinguish one touch from two on his finger pads.

Following the same procedure, test your patient's arms, legs, and torso.

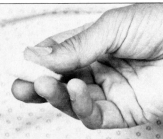

9 To test your patient's point localization ability, touch each hand with an applicator stick, as the nurse is doing here. Ask your patient to tell you where he feels the applicator.

Repeat the test on other parts of his body. Note the results.

10 Now you'll want to test Mr. Boyle's ability to discriminate textures. To do this, place a piece of cotton in his right hand. Ask him to identify the substance. Repeat the procedure with other distinct textures, such as a paper towel or waxed paper.

Then, use the same procedure to test his left hand.

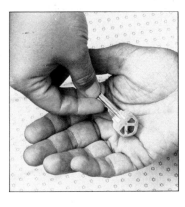

11 Next, test your patient's stereognostic function by asking him to identify small common objects; for example, a key, and coins (nickel, dime, and quarter). To do this, place the key in the palm of his right hand. Ask him to identify it. If all's well, he should easily manipulate the key and correctly identify it. Repeat this procedure with the remaining test items. Then, using the same procedure, test his left hand.

Assessment

Assessing your
patient's sensory system continued

12 To assess Mr. Boyle's number identification ability, grasp his right hand, palm facing up. Using the blunt end of a pen or pencil, write a large number or letter on his palm. Can he correctly identify it? If so, his graphesthesia sensation is intact. Follow this procedure on his left palm and compare the results.

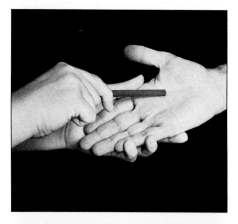

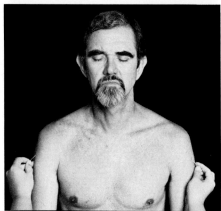

13 Finally, you'll need to determine whether your patient exhibits an extinction phenomenon. To do this, you'll need two pins. Simultaneously touch identical locations on each of your patient's arms. Ask your patient to tell you where you have touched him. If he says both arms, consider this a normal response. If he answers one arm, ask which arm and have him point to where on his arm you've touched him.

Repeat this test on other corresponding areas on opposite sides of his body.

Document all tests performed and responses in your notes. If your patient responds normally in those tests for the primary forms of sensation, but exhibits abnormal responses in the discriminatory tests, suspect parietal lobe involvement.

How to use
a dermatome chart

The two figures on this page illustrate the segmental distribution of spinal nerves that transmit pain, temperature, and touch from the skin to the spinal cord.

As you assess your patient's sensory function, refer to this chart to document the specific area tested, as well as the test results.

For example, let's say your patient can't differentiate between hot and cold test tubes placed at the umbilicus level. Using the dermatome chart, you'd document the test result as a loss of temperature sensation in the T_{10} to T_{11} areas.

Remember, a dermatome chart's segmental levels may vary slightly. So when documenting your patient's test results always use your hospital's chart.

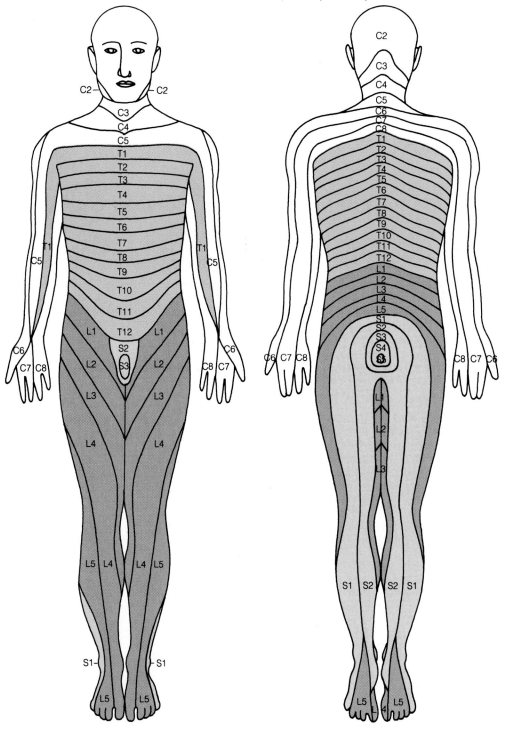

Identifying testing hammers

Hammers used for neurologic reflex testing come in a variety of shapes and styles. Four different models are shown below.

As you know, some hammers have removable accessories in addition to the head, such as a pin or brush. These models are called neurologic hammers.

Other models come equipped with just a hammer head and are called reflex hammers.

When choosing a hammer, always select a model that fits comfortably, and moves freely in your hand. Both considerations are essential to ensure accurate test results.

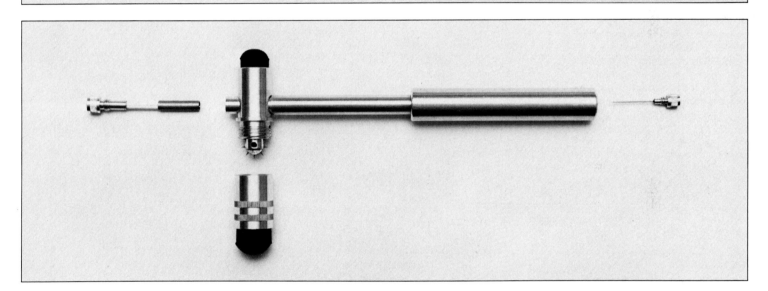

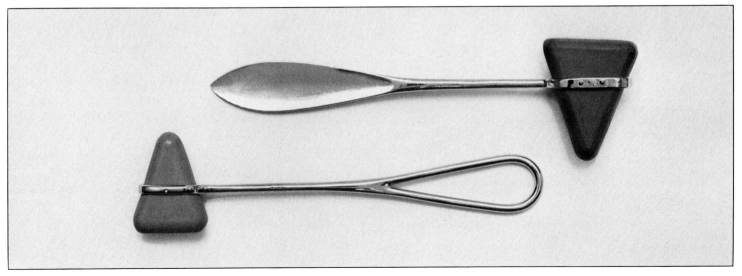

Assessment

Assessing your patient's reflexes

1 *To complete Mr. Boyle's neurologic assessment, you'll need to evaluate the rapidity and strength of three types of reflexes: deep, superficial, and pathologic. Remember, always apply the same stimuli on each side of your patient's body with the same degree of force. Here's how to proceed:*

First, obtain a moderately sharp object, for example, a key or applicator stick, and a reflex hammer. (Make sure the object isn't sharp enough to break the skin.) Then, explain each test to your patient. Encourage him to relax each part of his body as you test it.

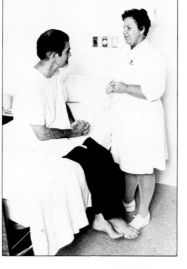

2 Now you're ready to test your patient's deep tendon reflexes. Begin with his biceps reflex. Slightly flex his right elbow. Then, with your thumb pressed firmly against his biceps muscle tendon, hold your patient's elbow.

[Inset] Keeping the reflex hammer held loosely between your thumb and fingers (allowing it to swing freely), strike your thumb. Expect your patient's biceps muscle to contract, flexing his arm at the elbow.

Repeat the test on your patient's left bicep.

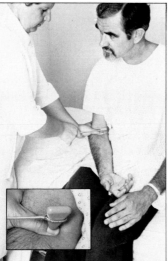

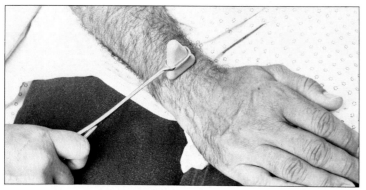

3 To assess your patient's supinator longus reflex, have him rest his forearm in his lap. His palm should be facing down. With the wide end of the reflex hammer, strike the radius, usually located about 1″ to 2″ (2.5 to 5 cm) above the wrist. If all's well, your patient's forearm will flex, so his palm turns upward.
Repeat the test on his other radial muscle.

4 Next, assess your patient's triceps reflex. To do this, have him flex his arm at the elbow. Then, hold his arm at the wrist. With the reflex hammer, strike the triceps tendon directly over his elbow. The triceps muscle should contract, extending your patient's arm at the elbow. Repeat the test on his other elbow.

[Inset] If your patient can't relax enough to produce an accurate triceps reflex, hold his arm to the side. Tell him to relax his arm, then strike the tendon.

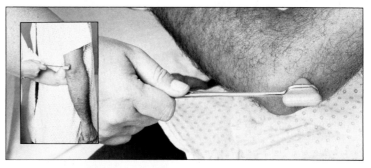

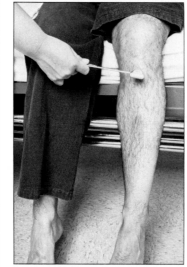

5 Test your patient's patellar reflex by using the reflex hammer to briskly strike his patellar tendon just below the patella. Expect to see knee extension, causing his leg to swing forward.
Repeat the test on his other knee.

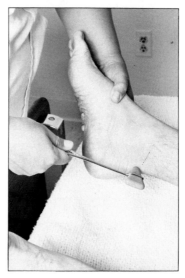

6 The last deep reflex to assess is the Achilles tendon reflex. To do this, hold your patient's right foot with your left hand. Gently rotate his foot outward and strike his Achilles tendon with the reflex hammer. As you do, watch the plantar flexion of his ankle. Then, observe how quickly the muscle relaxes after contraction. If this relaxation period is slowed, suspect hypothyroidism.
Repeat the test on his left Achilles tendon.

7 Now you're ready to assess Mr. Boyle's superficial reflexes. First, have him lie on the bed in a supine position. His legs should be slightly flexed at the knees. Tell him to keep both arms at his side during the test. Expose his abdomen.

Now, instruct your patient to exhale. As he does, gently pull the applicator stick across his upper right abdomen, from the outer side toward his umbilicus (see top photo). Normally, the umbilicus will move up and toward the area being touched. If your patient has an upper or lower motor neuron disturbance, his abdominal reflex may be absent. Repeat the test on his upper left abdomen (lower photo).

Then, test both sides of his lower abdomen. Expect the umbilicus to move down.

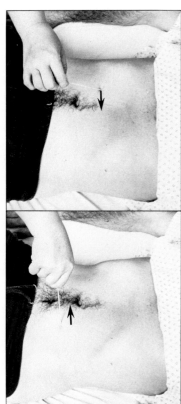

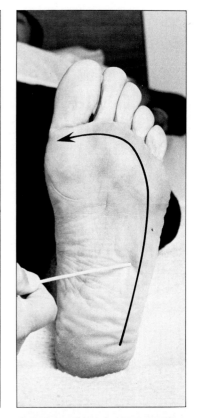

9 To test your patient's plantar reflex, lightly scratch the outer lateral aspect of his foot, from the heel up. If everything's okay, his toes will curl downward. Then, repeat the test on his other foot.

10 Suppose, in response to the plantar reflex test, his great toe dorsiflexes (inset) and his other toes fan out. This reflex is considered pathologic and is known as the Babinski sign. It indicates pyramidal tract disease. Other responses which may occur simultaneously and help to confirm the Babinski sign are: dorsiflexion of the ankle, and flexion of the knee and hip.

To confirm the Babinski sign, repeat the plantar reflex test on the foot exhibiting the sign. But, never apply too much pressure with your stimuli. This action may cause a voluntary withdrawal in a normal patient, which may be confused with a pathologic neurologic response.

Document everything in your notes.

Note: In some hospitals, a grading system, ranging from 0 (no reflex) to 4++++ (hyperactive) is used to document a patient's reflexes. Grades 2++ to 3+++ indicate normal reflexes.

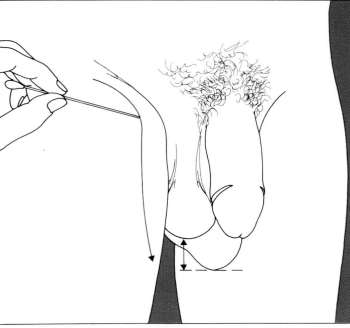

8 Now, if your patient's male, you'll also need to test the cremasteric reflex. Gently draw the stick down the upper portion of his right inner thigh, as shown here. Expect the right cremasteric muscle to contract and the right testicle to rise slightly. Absence of the cremasteric reflex may be present in upper and lower motor neuron disturbances. Then, repeat the test on your patient's left side.

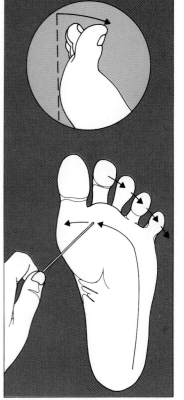

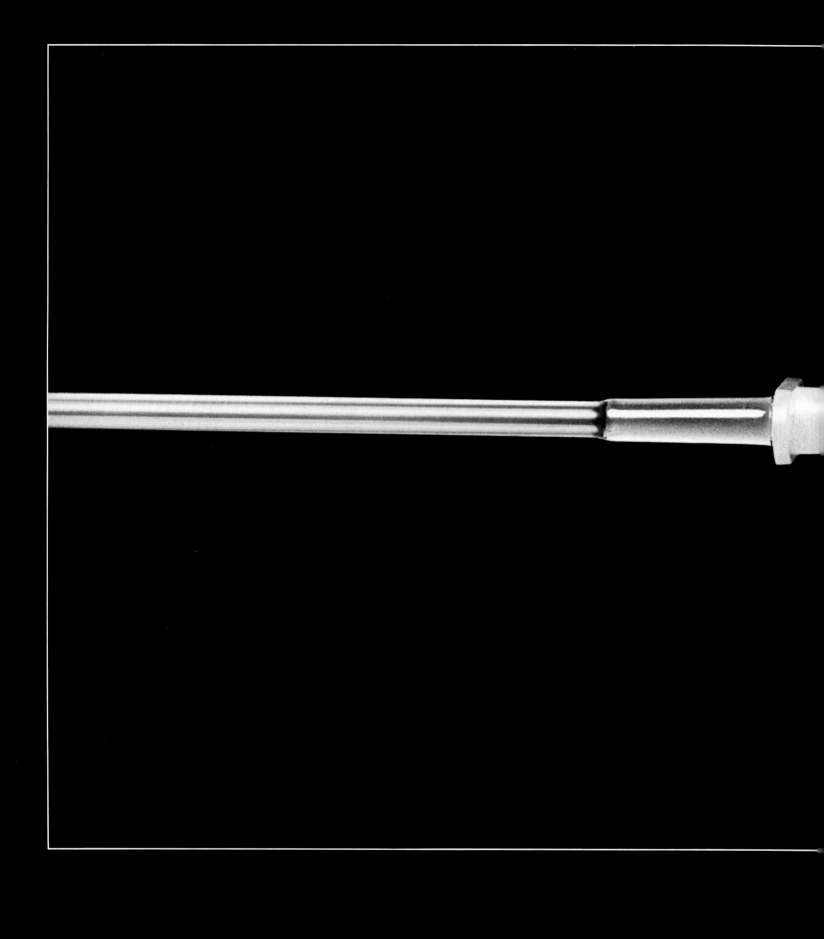

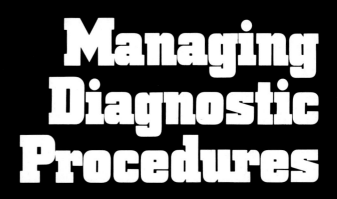

Managing Diagnostic Procedures

Noninvasive tests

Invasive tests

Noninvasive tests

Ever wonder what electroencephalography, echoencephalography, and a computerized tomography (CT) scanning have in common? All are noninvasive neurologic testing procedures.

But these procedures differ in various ways. For example, an electroencephalograph records the brain's electrical activity through a system of leads and electrodes. Echoencephalography helps determine ventricular size and detect cerebral midline shifts using ultrasonic waves. CT scanning, on the other hand, examines horizontal slices of the brain through a system of X-rays and scintillation detectors. We'll show you the equipment and how it works.

In the following pages, you'll learn about noninvasive testing procedures. More importantly, you'll learn how to reduce your patient's fear and anxiety by preparing him properly.

Getting your patient ready for testing

Let's say the doctor orders skull and spinal X-rays, and a computerized tomography (CT) scan for your patient. These test results will help the doctor identify or rule out a neurologic disorder. You can help prepare your patient for these tests. Here's how:

• Explain why the doctor's ordered the tests, if possible.
• Review the testing procedure with your patient.
• Describe the equipment he'll see in the testing area. Keep in mind that the large, unfamiliar machinery may make him nervous.
• Explain that he'll receive only a small amount of radiation during the CT scan and X-ray procedures. Assure him that the procedures are entirely safe. Tell him that others in the room may wear lead aprons to shield themselves from radiation because they're exposed to several X-rays or CT scans each day.
• If your patient's female, ask her when she had her last menstrual period. Is there a chance she's pregnant? If so, ask the technician to shield her

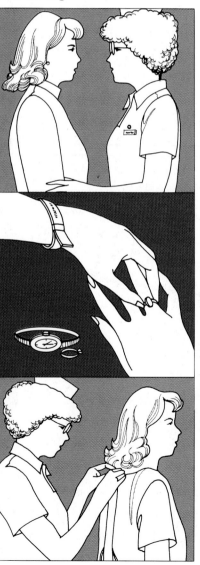

uterus; advise the patient of this special precaution.
• For a skull or spinal X-ray, warn your patient that the X-ray plate will feel cold.
• Encourage questions and answer them completely and honestly.
• Ask your patient to remove dentures, jewelry, and any other metal objects above his waist, and explain why. (Metal objects will show up on X-rays and may look like abnormalities.) For a CT scan, your patient will also have to remove such dense objects as a hearing aid, glasses, contact lenses, pierced earrings, a bracelet, or a necklace. (Metal or dense objects may block the X-rays.)
• Help your patient into a hospital or X-ray gown with a tie fastener. To protect his privacy and help him feel more comfortable, tell him he can also wear pajama bottoms with a tie fastener.

Note: Never give your patient a gown or pajama bottoms with metal snaps, because snaps show up on X-rays.

Document all patient teaching and preparation in your nurses' notes.

Performing diagnostic procedures: some tips

Whenever a patient's scheduled for noninvasive testing, it's your responsibility to make sure he's prepared properly. Whether you accompany him to the testing area or arrange for a co-worker to assume patient responsibility during the test, you'll need the following information to complete his chart: patient's name and room number, test being performed, pertinent medical history, baseline assessment data, and your name and title.

Remember: The patient's chart will accompany him to the testing area.

Now, here are some other important guidelines to remember when preparing your patient:
• Obtain a signed consent form from the patient or his family prior to the test and sedative administration.
• Administer a sedative 1 hour before the test, as ordered.
• Administer routine medications as ordered.
• Make sure the patient's neurologic and physical baseline data is accurate and up-to-date.
• Following the doctor's orders, withhold food and oral fluids before the test.
• Ensure correct patient identity by checking his identification band with the Kardex or doctor's orders.
• Provide your patient with a hospital gown and pajama bottoms (if needed) for the test. Make sure the gown and pajamas have tie fasteners.
• Before the transfer, provide any special care the patient needs; for example, administering oxygen, giving I.V. feedings, or applying traction.
• Ask him to urinate before he leaves your unit.
• Assess the patient's tolerance to the testing position. Notify the doctor if you suspect a problem.

Document all your preparations in your nurses' notes.

Learning about skull and spinal X-rays

The doctor's ordered skull and spinal X-rays as a part of your patient's neurologic workup. Studying these noninvasive test results will help him identify relationships between injured bone and tissue, and surrounding structures. The results of these studies will help him establish a diagnosis or rule out the following conditions:
• head, neck, and spinal trauma, including fractures
• calcifications, such as an old or chronic subdural hematoma, or a tumor
• structural displacement caused by a tumor or other space-occupying lesion; for example, a pineal body shift
• degenerative changes, including bone erosions, and arthritis
• other abnormalities, such as major vascular changes or congenital anomalies.

Prepare your patient for X-ray by explaining the procedure and reassuring him that the X-rays will not be painful. Next, consider the following special precautions you must observe when a problem is suspected to be neurologic:
• Ensure your patient's safety during his transfer to X-ray. Do this, once he's on the stretcher, by securing the safety belts and raising the side rails.
• Tell your patient he must remain motionless during the X-ray. Ease any muscle spasms or pain he has by administering an analgesic or antispasmodic, as ordered. Quiet the restless or uncooperative patient by administering a sedative, as ordered.
• Make sure your patient's spinal cord and neck remain immobilized to prevent further injury or vascular disruption to his spinal

cord. For example, if your patient's wearing a cervical collar, use sandbags or a head brace to help stabilize his head and neck. If your patient's in traction, maintain proper traction at all times. Do not change his traction angle or direction unless ordered by the doctor. *Note:* If the patient can't be transferred, the doctor will order a portable X-ray.
• Tell the X-ray technicians not to remove your patient's dressings (if he has any), and to notify you if any dressings come loose.
• Accompany your patient to the X-ray department in the following cases: if he has respiratory distress, a suspected spinal cord injury, an altered state of consciousness, a suspected cerebellar tonsillar herniation, or if he's an ICU neurologic patient.

Preparing your patient for electroencephalography

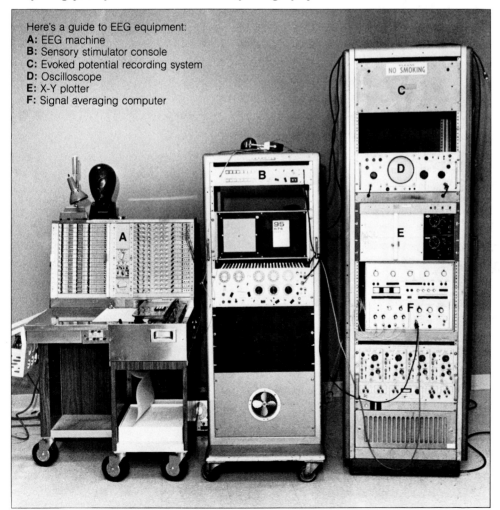

Here's a guide to EEG equipment:
A: EEG machine
B: Sensory stimulator console
C: Evoked potential recording system
D: Oscilloscope
E: X-Y plotter
F: Signal averaging computer

Ever care for a patient scheduled for electroencephalography? If you have, then you know how important it is to help him understand the test procedure.

Explain the importance of the EEG machine, lead wires, and electrodes. Tell him that the technician will attach from 17 to 21 contact electrodes to his unshaven scalp. But assure him that the EEG machine only records brain activity; it doesn't discharge electricity into the brain. It can't read minds or indicate mental or emotional stability.

Be sure your patient understands that he'll be placed in a quiet room during the test. Tell him this is so his brain will respond only to its inner workings and not any outside noise.

Here are some additional guidelines:
• Make sure the patient's hair is clean, combed smoothly over his head, and free of any colorings, sprays, and creams. This ensures proper electrode placement. If contact electrodes are used, your patient may wash his hair immediately after the test. However, if needle electrodes are used, he must wait 48 hours.
• Withhold stimulants, such as coffee, tea, and cola (if patient's not already on a stimulant-restricted diet).
• Advise the EEG technician of any electrical devices the patient has in place; for example, a ventilator, cardiac monitor, or hypothermia blanket. Tell the technician which devices may be disconnected (if any) during the procedure.
• Document all patient teaching and preparation in your nurses' notes.

Noninvasive tests

Understanding electroencephalography

1 *You probably know that the brain's made up of millions of nerve cells. These nerve cells give off varying degrees of electrical energy which stimulate and activate the brain and nervous system. The electroencephalograph (EEG) machine translates this electrical energy into waveforms on a viewing screen or paper readout.*

How does the EEG transmit electrical activity to a screen or readout? This photo shows a technician applying a series of electrodes to a patient's unshaven scalp. An electrode, which conducts electricity, detects electrical impulses generated by nerve cells in the brain. The illustrations below show electrode placement on the scalp.

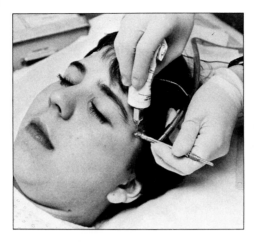

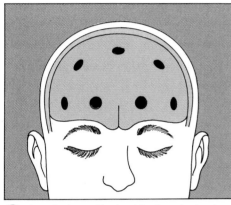

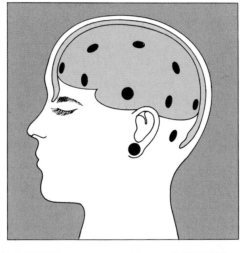

2 Lead wires attached to the electrodes transmit these impulses to the EEG machine.

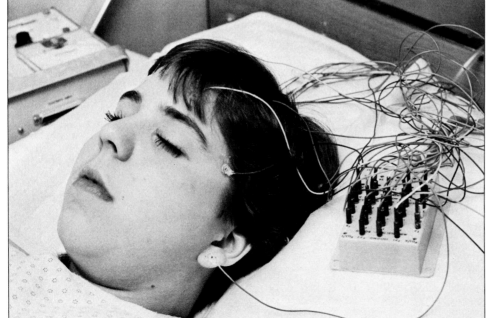

3 Let's say a nerve cell that's located near an electrode fires. The electrode will send this message through the lead wire to the EEG monitor.

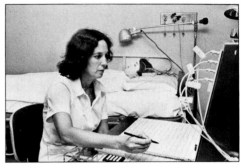

4 Almost immediately, you'll see a slight peak in the machine's screen and paper readout (see photos below). And, if several nerve cells fire at one time, the peak will appear higher. But when nerve cells stay quiet for a few seconds, you'll note a flat horizontal line on the screen. In other words, the height, shape, and amount of peaks in the waveform correspond to the amount of nerve cells firing at any given time.

But remember, an EEG waveform reflects overall electrical activity patterns, not the pattern or behavior of any single neuron.

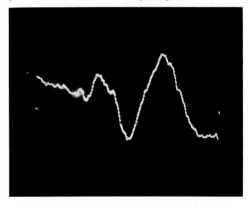

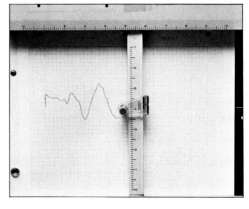

Reading electroencephalograms (EEGs)

Of course, interpreting EEG waveforms is primarily the responsibility of the doctor or EEG technician, but you can learn to recognize and understand normal waveforms. Then, you can compare your patient's waveforms to these and detect possible abnormalities.

As you know, by studying variations in EEG waveforms, the doctor or technician may be able to do the following:
- identify and localize space-occupying lesions
- identify and localize seizure foci
- diagnose brain death.

To read an EEG correctly, you must first familiarize yourself with the basic waveforms shown below. *Note:* They're listed in frequency order from fastest to slowest.

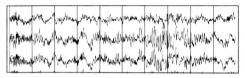

Beta waveforms indicate normal intense nervous system activity when a patient's awake (with his eyes open), and is alert and attentive. They occur at a rate of 18 to 30 per second in the cerebrum's frontal and central regions.

Alpha waveforms indicate normal alert brain activity when a patient's awake (with his eyes closed), and is relaxed and nonattentive. They occur at a rate of 8 to 12 per second in the parietal, occipital, and posterior parts of the temporal lobe.

Theta waveforms indicate emotional stress or drowsiness in adults. They occur at a rate of 4 to 7 per second.

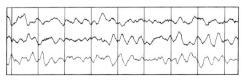

Delta waveforms indicate deep sleep or a serious brain disorder. They occur at a rate of less than 3½ per second.

Understanding echoencephalography

1 *How familiar are you with echoencephalography? As you know, this noninvasive procedure uses ultrasonic waves to help determine cerebral midline shifts and ventricular size. And keep in mind that increased ventricular size and a cerebral midline shift may indicate a rapidly expanding intracranial lesion.*

To perform the procedure, a doctor or skilled technician will place the machine's ultrasonic transducer on your patient's skull at the temporoparietal region, as shown. The transducer acts as a transmitter of ultrasonic waves and a receiver of a returning echo.

2 Now, the doctor will study the oscilloscope image. As he does, he'll systematically angle the transducer to direct ultrasonic waves to the cerebral midline structures, especially the third ventricle's lateral wall.

Wondering why the transducer's placed at the temporoparietal region? Because this location provides an acoustical window that avoids bone tissue. (You'll remember that ultrasound travels poorly through bone tissue.)

3 As you know, the cerebral midline structures will return an echo patttern on the oscilloscope. These responses, called M-echos, are also recorded permanently on film (see photo).

If your patient is scheduled for echoencephalography, be sure to review this procedure with him. Assure him that echoencephalography's safe and painless. And to ensure test accuracy, remind him to keep his head motionless during the procedure.

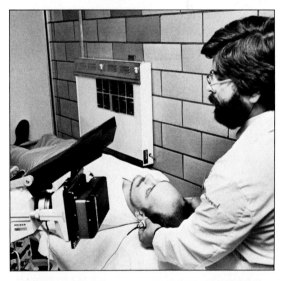

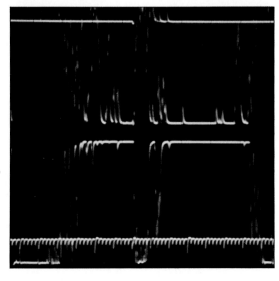

Noninvasive tests

Getting acquainted with the computerized tomography (CT) scanner

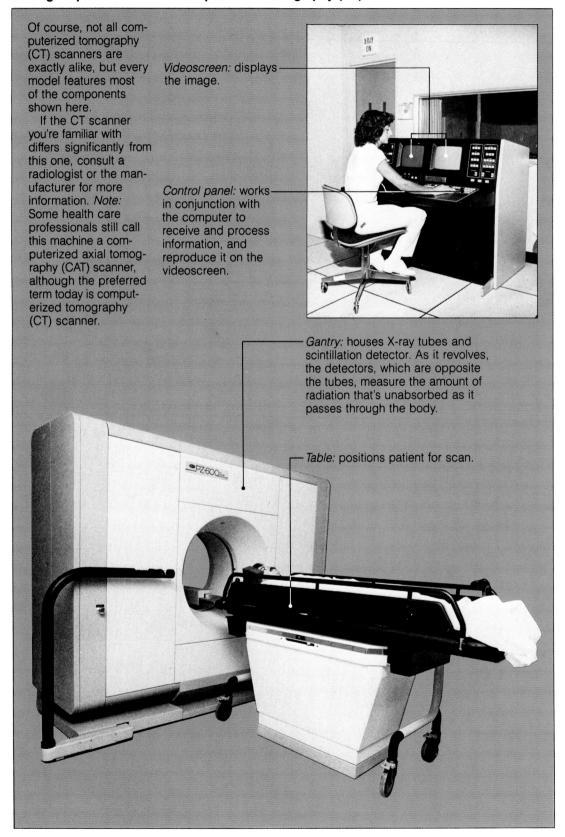

Of course, not all computerized tomography (CT) scanners are exactly alike, but every model features most of the components shown here.

If the CT scanner you're familiar with differs significantly from this one, consult a radiologist or the manufacturer for more information. *Note:* Some health care professionals still call this machine a computerized axial tomography (CAT) scanner, although the preferred term today is computerized tomography (CT) scanner.

Videoscreen: displays the image.

Control panel: works in conjunction with the computer to receive and process information, and reproduce it on the videoscreen.

Gantry: houses X-ray tubes and scintillation detector. As it revolves, the detectors, which are opposite the tubes, measure the amount of radiation that's unabsorbed as it passes through the body.

Table: positions patient for scan.

Preparing your patient for a computerized tomography (CT) scan

The doctor will order a computerized tomography (CT) scan of your patient's brain or spinal cord to help detect: calcifications; structural disorders, such as space-occupying lesions and tumors; and other abnormalities; for example, infarctions.

Important: CT scans are used to examine almost all bodily parts.

How does a CT scan work? A narrrow X-ray beam examines horizontal sections of the brain, cranium, or spinal cord (depending on the type of scan ordered). This X-ray beam, along with a system of scintillation detectors and a computer, produce a well-defined gray scale image on a videoscreen and Polaroid® film. By discriminating minute tissue density variations, the CT scan can help the doctor confirm a diagnosis. It can also help you assess a patient's condition, and plan appropriate nursing care.

In some cases, the doctor may wish to enhance tissue density by administering contrast dye I.V. The dye accumulates in masses or lesions (except in areas of poor blood supply) and helps him to see an area for minutes—rather than seconds.

What role do you play in the CT scan procedure? Your first job is to prepare your patient properly (see the guidelines on page 44). The day before, explain the procedure, its purpose, and the equipment your patient can expect to see. Assure him that the procedure's painless. Stress that he must stay motionless during the scan. Any movement, even a sneeze, will blur the image.

Tell your patient that although he may be alone in the scanner room, he can use the two-way intercom to talk to the technician or radiologist during the procedure. Also, tell him that the clicking noises he'll hear

Learning about a computerized tomography (CT) scan

during the scan are normal and indicate the scanner's operating properly.

Is your patient scheduled for a dye scan? If so, explain that when the dye enters his system, he may feel flushed and have a metallic taste in his mouth.

Then, follow these guidelines, as ordered by the doctor:

• Withhold solid foods for 2 hours prior to the scan. This precaution helps avoid nausea or vomiting that may follow a dye scan.

• Ask patient about his allergy history (especially to shellfish and iodine), and any other condition, such as asthma, that may cause him to react to the dye. Remember, iodine is contained in the contrast dye.

• Obtain a signed consent form and attach the form to the patient's chart.
About 1 hour before the CT scan, be sure to follow these guidelines:

• Comb your patient's hair smoothly over his head.

• Arrange for the patient to be transferred to the CT scan area. Make sure the patient's chart accompanies him to the scan area.

• Administer a sedative, if ordered by the doctor.

Suppose your patient had a dye scan. After the scan, look for signs and symptoms of an immediate or delayed anaphylactic reaction, such as restlessness, flushed face, palpitations, respiratory distress, urticaria, nausea and vomiting, decreased blood pressure, and tachycardia. If you see any of these signs, notify the doctor immediately. Because the dye's hypertonic, it may cause diuresis, so encourage your patient to drink plenty of fluids.

Document all preparations in your nurses' notes.

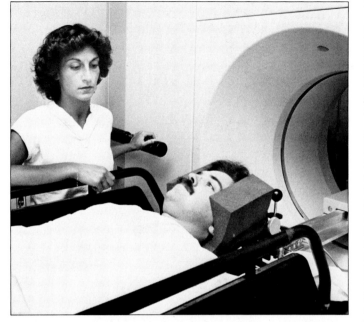

1 *Kent McLean is ready for his computerized tomography (CT) scan. You've prepared him mentally and physically. He's been transferred to your hospital's CT scan area. Do you know how the procedure progresses from here? If you're unsure, review these steps:*

First, the technician will review the CT scan procedure with Mr. McLean and show him how to operate the two-way intercom. She'll check to be sure Mr. McLean's consent form is signed. Then, she'll position Mr. McLean comfortably on the table inside the scanner's doughnut-like opening.
Next, the technician will secure the straps at Mr. McLean's head and waist. Doing so will help keep Mr. McLean motionless during the procedure.

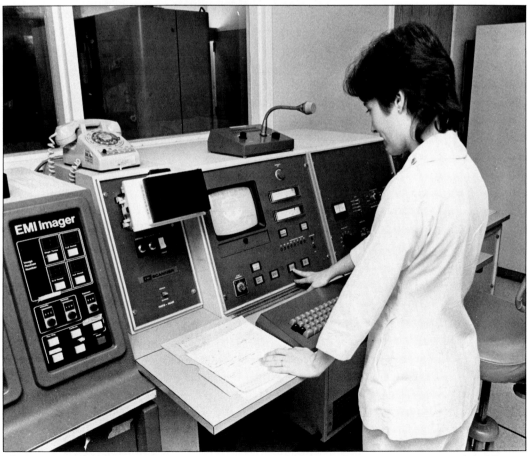

2 Knowing that the purpose of Mr. McLean's scan is to visualize cranial contents and structures, the radiologist programs the compu- ter. A planar image will appear on the videoscreen. This image shows the area and tissue to be scanned.

Noninvasive tests

3 Now the radiologist is ready to begin scanning. As the gantry revolves, detectors located in the gantry send thousands of radiation readings to the computer for processing and conversion into videoscreen and hard copy images. A scan of the first tissue slice comes into view on the screen.

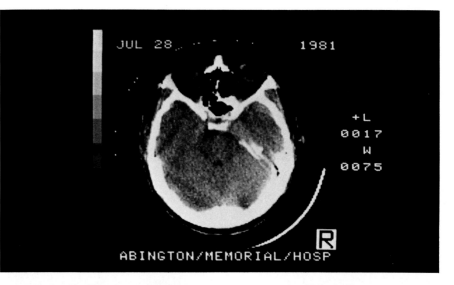

4 When the gantry's ready to scan the next tissue slice, you'll see the table move Mr. McLean into position.

The CT scanner will repeat this procedure six to eight times. When the predetermined area's represented on film (usually in 10 to 45 minutes) the scan's complete.

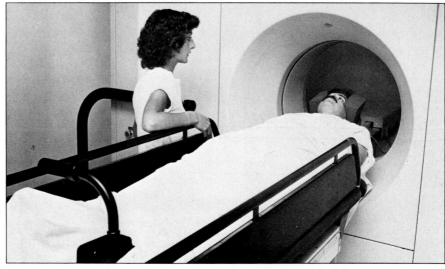

5 To provide a comparative scan for differential studies, Mr. McLean's doctor has ordered a dye scan. To prepare for this procedure, the technician will explain the dye scan to Mr. McLean. She'll ask him if he's allergic to shellfish or iodine or whether he has any conditions, such as asthma, which may cause him to react to the dye. Then, depending on hospital policy, she may ask Mr. McLean to sign another consent form.

Now the radiologist will insert the venipuncture line and infuse about 125 ml of dye I.V. at a fast rate. Then, she'll adjust the flow rate to slow, so an additional 125 ml of dye will infuse gradually during the scan.

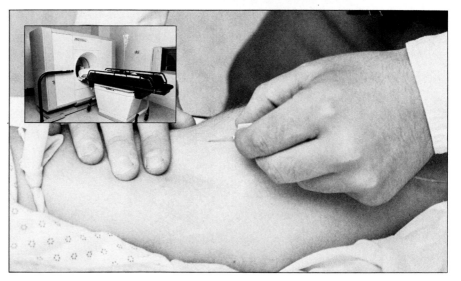

6 Is the radiologist administering the dye I.V. bolus? If so, she probably wants to see an immediate image on the videoscreen. Keep in mind, though, that I.V. bolus administration produces a short-lived image and may increase the possibility of a reaction.

Although serious allergic reactions to dye are rare, the nurse or technician will monitor Mr. McLean for signs and symptoms, such as nasal stuffiness, itching, and urticaria. If she notes any signs that suggest impending anaphylactic shock, the technician will notify the radiologist. The nurse will then administer diphenhydramine hydrochloride (Benadryl*), 50 mg I.V., as ordered.

Several hours after the dye scan, the radiologist may perform an additional non-dye scan. By comparing information from the two scans, she'll be able to read and interpret the results.

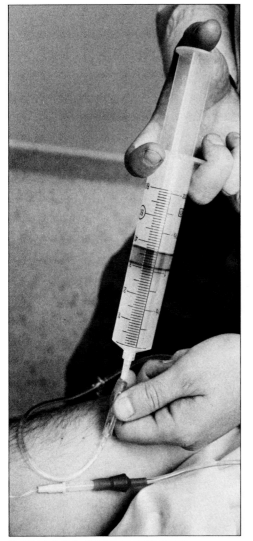

Reading a computerized tomography (CT) scan

After finishing a computerized tomography (CT) scan, the radiologist usually reads and interprets the results the same day. Sometimes he'll work from the screen image; at other times, he will use the hard copy image.

By comparing tissue densities on the screen or on hard copy, the radiologist can detect two types of abnormalities: anatomic (including changes in position, shape, and size, such as atrophy or hypertrophy); and attenuate (including changes in body part density, such as inflammation, edema, hemorrhage, neoplasms, blood clots, calcium deposits, tissue necrosis, cysts, and abscesses).

Finally, when his study's completed, he'll send a report and a copy of the scan to the patient's doctor.

Now, study the two scans on this page. They reflect 2 views taken during a CT scan of the brain. As you know, the scan identifies brain structures in the black to white spectrum according to densities. For example, structures with greater densities such as bone or hemorrhage show up as white.

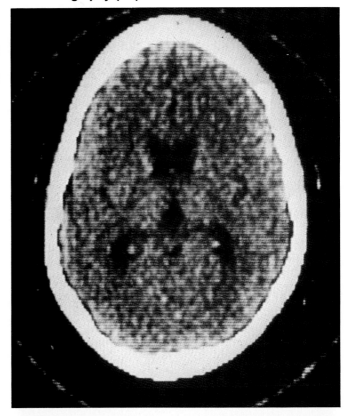

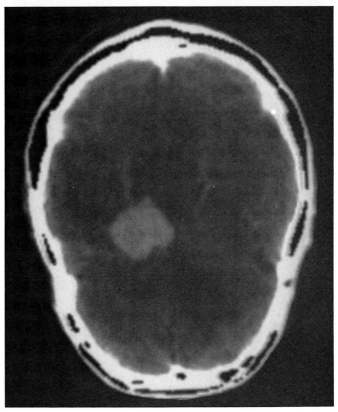

Invasive tests

Invasive neurologic testing can be frightening to both your patient and his family. So much depends on how well you prepare them before testing. For example, do you know how to explain a lumbar puncture to your patient? Your step-by-step details and emotional support will help him understand the procedure as well as what's expected of him. Or, in another case, your description of angiography and the importance of post-procedural bed rest may minimize complications.

Be completely prepared the next time you care for a patient scheduled for neurologic testing. Learn all you can about invasive testing procedures. Study the illustrations, charts, and photostories on these pages to find out how to properly prepare, monitor, and care for your patient before and after these test procedures.

Differentiating between invasive tests

During diagnostic testing, the doctor will probably order several invasive tests. Which tests will the doctor order? That depends on your patient's condition, the doctor's preference, and your hospital's equipment. This chart details how these tests differ.

Lumbar puncture

• A percutaneous puncture entering the spinal column's subarachnoid space at the vertebral interspace L_3-L_4 or L_4-L_5. A lumbar puncture is performed for cerebrospinal fluid (CSF) pressure measurement; withdrawal of a CSF specimen for analysis; and the introduction of contrast media for diagnostic tests.

Indications

• To reduce intracranial pressure (ICP) after a spontaneous hemorrhage, by releasing CSF.
• To help diagnose diffuse or disseminated infections of the nervous system or meninges; subarachnoid hemorrhage; or demyelinating diseases.
• To introduce anesthetic, antibiotics, or other therapeutic drugs into the area.
• To identify degree of subarachnoid blockage.

Special considerations

• Do not perform when increased ICP may be caused by an expanding lesion, such as a subdural hematoma after a head injury.
• Perform cautiously in patient with suspected spinal cord or brain tumor. Procedure may cause fatal cerebellar tonsillar herniation or compression of medulla.
• After the procedure, keep patient flat in bed for 4 to 6 hours. Encourage him to drink plenty of fluids.
• Observe puncture site for edema, hematoma, and CSF leakage.
• Perform a neurocheck, as ordered or indicated.

Pneumoencephalography

• Infusion of a gas such as air, nitrous oxide, or oxygen, through a lumbar or cisternal puncture. A series of X-rays taken during the infusion allows the doctor to visualize the ventricular system and meningeal spaces. In some hospitals, angiography and computerized tomography have replaced this test, but it remains a valuable diagnostic tool for certain types of lesions.

Indications

• To identify lesions by determining ventricular size, shape, and position.

Special considerations

• Administer medications as needed for headache, nausea, vomiting, diaphoresis, and dizziness.
• Keep patient flat in bed for 24 to 48 hours. Every 2 hours, change your patient's position from side to side.
• Unless your patient complains of nausea, encourage him to drink plenty of fluids and eat foods high in sodium. Doing so replaces CSF and promotes reabsorption of the infused air.
• Notify the doctor if you note increased ICP, seizures, shock, prolonged or intractable headache, nausea, vomiting, chills, or fever.

Myelography

• Infusion of dye or gas into spinal column's subarachnoid space through a lumbar puncture. A series of X-rays taken during the infusion allows the doctor to visualize the spinal column.

Indications

• To identify space-occupying lesions of the spinal cord.
• To help diagnose a herniated nucleus pulposus.

Special considerations

• Administer medications, as ordered, for headache, nausea, vomiting, diaphoresis, and dizziness.
• Keep patient in bed for 24 to 48 hours, as ordered. Elevate the head of his bed, as ordered.
• Perform a neurocheck, as ordered.
• Unless your patient feels nauseated, encourage him to drink plenty of fluids and eat foods high in sodium.
• Notify the doctor if you note increased ICP, seizures, shock, prolonged or intractable headache, nausea, vomiting, chills, or fever.

Cisternal puncture

Ventriculography

Angiography

Brain scan

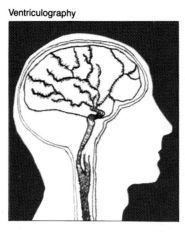
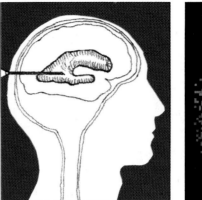
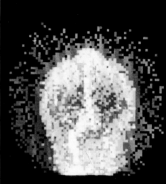

Cisternal puncture
• A puncture entering the subarachnoid space between the cerebellum and the medulla (cisterna magna) located between the first cervical lamina and the ridge of the foramen magnum. Insertion of a short, beveled needle allows for CSF pressure measurements; CSF withdrawal for analysis; and introduction of contrast media for diagnostic tests.
Indications
• Performed when a lumbar puncture's contraindicated or a subarachnoid block exists.
• To reduce ICP.
• To help diagnose: diffuse or disseminated infections of the nervous system or meninges; a subarachnoid hemorrhage; or a demyelinating disease.
Special considerations
• Assess patient frequently for signs and symptoms of cerebellar tonsillar medullary herniation, such as nuchal rigidity, motor paralysis, jackknife spasticity, hyperactive deep tendon reflexes in involved limb, medullary collapse, or circulatory collapse.

Ventriculography
• Infusion of air or dye into the lateral ventricle through a puncture in the skull. A series of X-rays taken during the infusion allows the doctor to visualize the ventricular and meningeal vascular systems. Performed when a lumbar or cisternal puncture is contraindicated to relieve elevated ICP.
Indications
• To ensure ventricular system patency.
• To establish ventricular drainage.
• To identify and localize lesions and tumors.
• To identify cerebral anomalies.
Special considerations
• Prepare patient for surgery, as ordered. In many cases, a craniotomy follows this procedure.
• If a ventricular tube must remain in place after the procedure, maintain a sterile closed system.
• Notify the doctor if you note hemorrhage, respiratory distress, increased ICP, seizures, hypovolemic shock, prolonged headache, nausea, vomiting, chills, or fever.
• Be sure to have a lumbar puncture tray at the patient's bedside in case a lumbar puncture is indicated to relieve sudden increased CSF pressure.
• Administer medications as ordered, for headache, nausea, vomiting, diaphoresis, and dizziness.
• Keep patient flat in bed for 24 to 48 hours. Elevate patient's head 15 to 20 degrees. Every 2 hours, change your patient's position from side to side.
• Encourage your patient to drink plenty of fluids, and eat foods high in sodium, if he can.

Cerebral angiography
Infusion of dye through a catheter directly or indirectly into the arterial system. A series of X-rays taken during the infusion allows the doctor to visualize the cerebral vasculature.

Indications
• To identify cerebral circulatory anomalies, such as a subdural hematoma, epidural hematoma, massive intracranial lesion, cerebral edema, carotid-cavernous sinus fistula, or aneurysm.
Special considerations
• Keep patient in bed for 24 to 48 hours, as ordered.
• Monitor vital signs and perform a neurocheck, as ordered.
• Notify the doctor if you note puncture site hemorrhage, hematoma, signs of increased ICP, seizures, nausea, vomiting, chills, or fever.
• Apply ice packs to puncture site, as ordered.
• Check patient's circulation, as well as his ability to move.
• Encourage patient to drink plenty of fluids, unless he feels nauseated.
• Administer medications, as ordered, for headache, nausea, vomiting, diaphoresis, and dizziness.

Brain scan
Infusion of a radioactive isotope I.V. A scintillation scanner measures the isotope's radiation emission and transmits a brain image onto a videoscreen. The isotope will accumulate in abnormal or damaged brain tissue.
Indications
• To identify intracranial diseases, such as gliomas and astrocytomas.
• To detect any remaining or spreading malignant tumors, following radiotherapy, chemotherapy, or a craniotomy.
Special considerations
• Assure your patient that the procedure is hazard-free. The isotope contains less radioactivity than X-rays.
• Tell the patient that repeat scans are usually necessary. Inform him that follow-up scans help the doctor monitor progress.

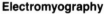

Electromyography
Insertion of a surface needle or electrode into a skeletal muscle. An oscilloscope records subsequent electrical activity for audio and visual analysis.
Indications
• To identify and localize lower motor neuron diseases, such as muscular dystrophy.
• To assess the status of peripheral nerve reinnervation.
Special considerations
• Advise patient to expect some muscle tenderness after the test.
• Administer ice packs, as necessary.

Electromyography

Invasive tests

Learning about a lumbar puncture

You probably know a number of reasons why the doctor performs a lumbar puncture. But do you know when he shouldn't? For example, suppose your patient has increasing intracranial pressure (ICP) from a suspected expanding lesion. In this situation, a lumbar puncture may be fatal. Why? Because cerebrospinal fluid (CSF) withdrawn for lab analysis decreases intracranial pressure and gives the lesion more space to expand. In some patients, this expansion may cause cerebellar tonsillar herniation, medullary compression—and death.

Is your patient scheduled for ventriculography, pneumoencephalography, or myelography? If so, the doctor will introduce air, gas, or dye into your patient's ventricle or subarachnoid space. He'll perform these tests to locate tumors, ensure ventricular patency, and identify structural abnormalities.

What are your responsibilities during these invasive procedures? Patient preparation for one. To find out more about these tests, how they differ, and how to prepare your patient properly, read the pages that follow.

Performing a lumbar puncture

1 *In this photostory, we'll show you how to assist the doctor with a lumbar puncture.*

· First, gather the equipment you'll need: a sterile lumbar puncture tray, two pairs of sterile gloves, grease or wax pencil, paper cup, and a face mask for the doctor (optional).

Then, explain the procedure to your patient. Tell him he'll probably feel pressure during the procedure, but only for a few minutes. Assure him that the doctor will anesthetize the puncture site before he performs the procedure.

Now, follow these steps:

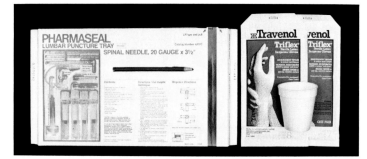

2 Have your patient lie on his side and bring his knees up toward his head, as shown here. Be sure his spine's curved and his back is at the edge of the bed, close to the doctor. This position opens the spaces between the vertebrae, allowing the doctor to insert the spinal needle more easily. Instruct your patient not to move or twist his spine during the procedure.

Note: Some doctors may prefer the patient to be positioned differently.

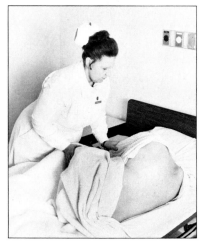

Preparing your patient for a lumbar puncture

Your patient, Tom Boyle, watches as you open the lumbar puncture tray on his bedside table. He knows the doctor has scheduled him for a lumbar puncture, but he suddenly remembers little of what you've told him about the procedure. He appears nervous and scared. "Will it hurt?" he asks, anxiously. How do you answer?

Tell him again that in the beginning of the procedure he'll feel slight discomfort as the doctor injects the local anesthetic. But assure him that after he receives this drug he'll feel only slight pressure in his lower back. Explain again how the lumbar puncture's performed and how it can help the doctor diagnose his condition. But, don't stop there. Make your explanation of the lumbar puncture procedure clearer by reviewing some basics about the brain and spinal cord (see pages 8 to 15).

The questions and answers that follow will give you an idea of some

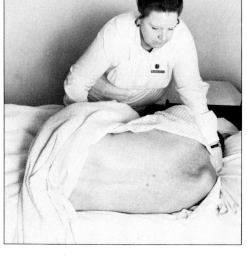

3 Suppose your patient can't hold this position. Then, place one hand behind his neck and the other hand behind his knees, and pull gently, as the nurse is doing here. Help him hold this position throughout the procedure.

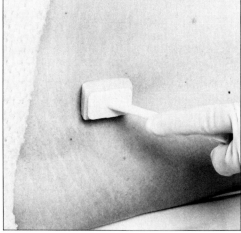

4 Now, using aseptic technique, open the lumbar puncture tray.

Then, prep the puncture site with an antiseptic solution, such as povidone-iodine. Work from the inside out, as shown here. Repeat this procedure three times.

Nursing tip: Each time you cleanse the puncture site, use a new swab or sponge to prevent contamination.

information your patient may want to know. Study the dialogue carefully. And remember, if you don't know the answer to any of your patient's questions, tell him you'll get the information for him. Then, be sure you do.

Mr. Boyle: What is a lumbar puncture?

Your answer: The term refers to a needle inserted through the lumbar portion of the spinal column. Actually, the needle will be inserted between your vertebrae. By performing this procedure, the doctor can measure your cerebrospinal fluid (CSF) pressure and obtain CSF samples. He'll send these samples to the lab for analysis.

Mr. Boyle: Why is the doctor sending my cerebrospinal fluid to the lab?

Your answer: Laboratory tests tell the doctor the elements that make up your CSF. By knowing the number and type of cells, and how much glucose and protein is in your CSF, the doctor may be able to diagnose your condition.

Mr. Boyle: How does measuring my CSF pressure tell the doctor about my brain?

Your answer: By studying CSF pressure readings, the doctor may be able to identify what's happening in your brain. In some cases, CSF pressure readings help the doctor rule out specific problems.

Mr. Boyle: Will I have more than one lumbar puncture?

Your answer: Not at one time. But the doctor may want to perform another lumbar puncture at another time during your hospitalization. By studying the results, the doctor can monitor your condition.

Mr. Boyle: What do I do during the test?

Your answer: Lie on your side with your head tucked downward and your knees brought up close to your chest. Breathe normally and lie still.

Mr. Boyle: Will I be up and around after the procedure?

Your answer: No, the doctor will want you to lie flat in bed for 4 to 6 hours after the procedure. He'll also want you to drink plenty of fluids. These precautions help prevent a headache from CSF loss.

Of course, while you're lying in bed, you can watch television, listen to the radio, and see visitors. If you need a bedpan or anything else during this 4 to 6 hour period, use the call bell at the side of your bed to notify a nurse.

5 Encourage your patient to lie still as the doctor anesthetizes the area.

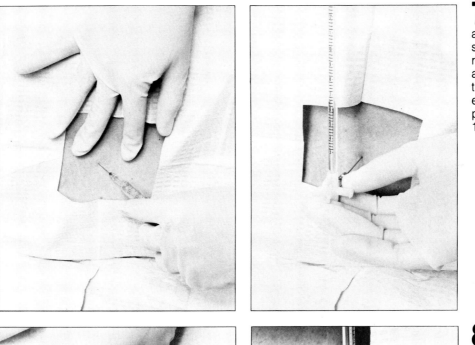

7 Now, the doctor attaches the stopcock and manometer to the spinal needle. Continue to reassure your patient, as the doctor measures the CSF pressure. If everything's okay, the pressure will be 60 to 180 mm of water.

6 Next, the doctor will insert the spinal needle in the vertebral interspace at the L_{3-4} or L_{4-5} level. When the doctor reaches the subarachnoid space, he'll remove the stylet and drain out a small amount of cerebrospinal fluid (CSF) to determine correct placement, as shown in this photo.

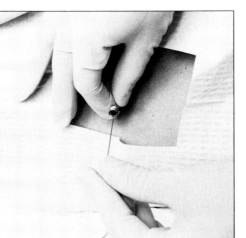

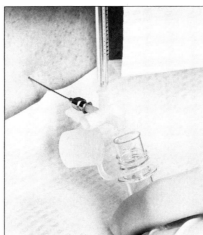

8 Next, the doctor will fill several tubes with cerebrospinal fluid.

After the doctor fills the first tube, he may hand you the capped tube. Keep the tube upright as you use a grease pencil to mark it No. 1 (unless it's been previously numbered). Then, place the tube in the paper cup.

Repeat this procedure with each tube, numbering them sequentially.

Invasive tests

Performing a lumbar puncture continued

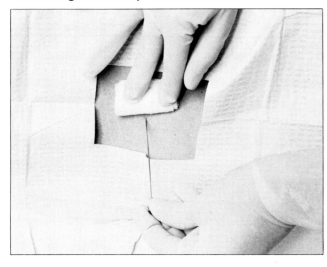

9 As the doctor withdraws the needle, apply direct pressure to the puncture site with a sterile gauze pad. After a few minutes, apply an adhesive bandage strip to the site.

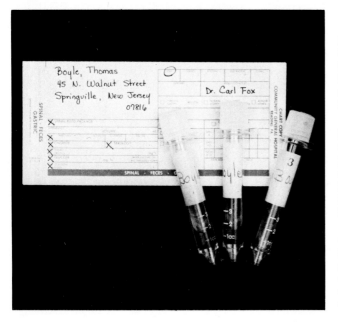

10 When the procedure's completed, position your patient flat in bed. Explain that he must remain in this position for 4 to 6 hours, (or as ordered), and that he may turn from side to side. Remaining flat may help prevent him from getting a headache from spinal fluid loss.
Note: Encourage your patient to drink plenty of fluids to help his body replace lost CSF.

11 Now, complete the necessary lab slips. If you're sending more than one slip, number them sequentially. Attach the slips to the specimen tubes and send the specimens to the lab immediately.

Perform a neurocheck on your patient, as ordered or indicated. Observe the puncture site for signs of edema, hematoma, and CSF leakage. If you see any of these, notify the doctor immediately.

Finally, document the procedure in your notes, including the pressure, color, consistency and amount of CSF removed, the patient's vital signs, and his tolerance to the procedure.

Assisting with Queckenstedt's test

When the doctor suspects your patient's subarachnoid space is occluded, he'll perform Queckenstedt's test. As you know, a subarachnoid space occlusion can be caused by a tumor, vertebral dislocation, or fracture. Do you know how to assist the doctor with this test? Here's how to proceed:
Note: You'll need to ask a co-worker for assistance.

First, the doctor will perform a lumbar puncture. Then, he'll attach the stopcock and manometer to the needle and take the initial cerebrospinal fluid (CSF) pressure reading.

The doctor will instruct you to apply even fingertip pressure to both of your patient's jugular veins (top photo). Have your co-worker tell you when 10 seconds has passed.

Quickly release the pressure you've been applying so the doctor can take the first CSF pressure reading (bottom photo). Then, with the co-worker timing and recording the results, the doctor will take a CSF pressure reading every 10 seconds. (See the next page for details on interpreting test results.)
Important: Closely monitor your patient for signs of increasing intracranial pressure (ICP) during Queckenstedt's test. This test may be hazardous, particularly in patients with increased ICP.

Finally, document the procedure, including ICP pressure readings and your patient's tolerance to the procedure, in your nurses' notes.

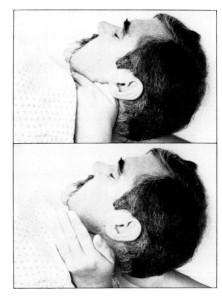

Interpreting Queckenstedt's test results

Does your patient have a subarachnoid space occlusion? He may, depending on his cerebrospinal fluid (CSF) pressure reading pattern. To find out, the doctor may perform Queckenstedt's test. Here's how to interpret the results:
• Rapidly rising CSF pressure reaching 100 to 300 ml of water from the initial pressure reading, which falls to the initial pressure reading within 30 seconds, means your patient's normal and free of any subarachnoid space occlusion.
• Slowly rising CSF pressure (or secondary rise) means your patient may have a partial subarachnoid space occlusion.
• No secondary rise in CSF pressure means your patient may have a total subarachnoid space occlusion.

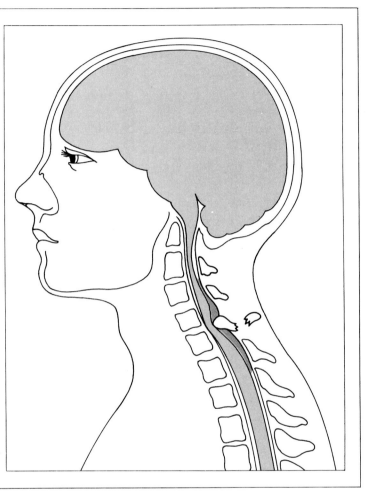

How to perform a cisternal puncture

As you probably know, the doctor will perform a cisternal puncture when a lumbar puncture's contraindicated. Like a lumbar puncture, a cisternal puncture is performed to measure and withdraw cerebrospinal fluid (CSF).

Wondering how to prepare your patient? First, shave the area from his occiput to his midcervical region, as ordered.

Now, position him at the edge of the bed (on his side), with a sandbag slipped under his head. This position will keep his cervical spine and head in line with the thoracic spine.

Note: Some doctors prefer that the patient be placed in a prone or lateral recumbent position with his head flexed and held in place by the nurse for this procedure.

Then, cleanse the area with an antiseptic solution, such as povidone-iodine.

At this point, the doctor will insert the spinal needle at the patient's cisterna magna. From here the doctor will follow the lumbar puncture procedure described on pages 54 to 56.

Remember, thoroughly document the procedure, and your patient's tolerance to it, in your nurses' notes.

What can cerebrospinal fluid (CSF) tell you?

Consider this: Several hours ago, the doctor performed a lumbar puncture on your patient. Now you're attaching the completed lab slip to your patient's chart. Wondering what these diagnostic test results mean?

Although interpreting results from cerebrospinal fluid (CSF) samples is the doctor's responsibility, you can learn to identify the characteristics of some common disorders. Use the chart below as a guide.

	Intracranial abscess	Intracranial tumor	Cerebral infarct	Subarachnoid hemorrhage	Acute bacterial meningitis
Pressure Normal range is from 60 to 180 mm water	• Elevated	• Elevated	• Elevated	• Readings vary from normal to extreme elevation	• Readings vary from moderate to extreme elevation
Appearance Normally clear	• Clear, but may be discolored if abscess ruptures	• Clear	• Usually clear	• Pink to red	• Clear to purulent
Cellular makeup Normal is 0 to 5 lymphocytes	• Amount varies from normal to increased	• Increased	• Slightly increased	• Increase in red and white blood cells	• Increase in white blood cells, usually between 10,000 to 50,000
Protein Normal is 15 to 45 mg per 100 ml	• Results vary from normal to increased	• Increased	• Slightly increased	• Increased	• Increased
Glucose Normal is 60% to 80% of true blood sugar; 40 to 80 mg per 100 ml	• Results vary from normal to decreased	• Normal	• Normal	• Results vary from normal to marked decrease	• Decreased

Invasive tests

Performing a myelogram

1 *Your patient, 29-year-old Dot Barry, is in the X-ray department for a myelogram. First, the technician will place the patient on the myelogram table. Then he'll open the myelogram tray, shown here.*

Note: In this photostory, the doctor will be infusing dye through a lumbar puncture.

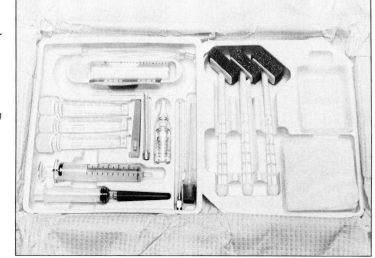

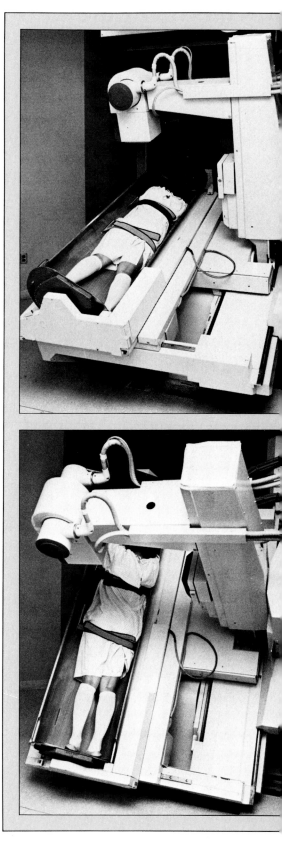

2 Now, the doctor will prep the puncture site and drape it with sterile towels, leaving a 4"x4" area exposed.

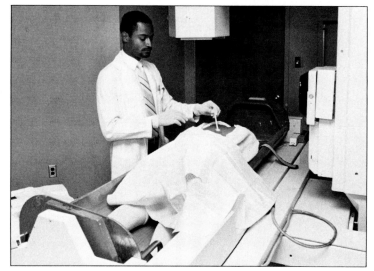

3 Next, the doctor will anesthetize the site and insert the lumbar puncture needle. After confirming entry into the subarachnoid space, he'll withdraw cerebrospinal fluid (CSF) and infuse the dye through the needle. When he's finished infusing the dye, he'll withdraw the needle and place an adhesive bandage strip over the insertion site.

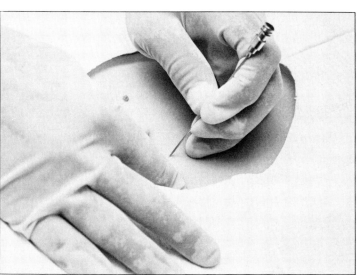

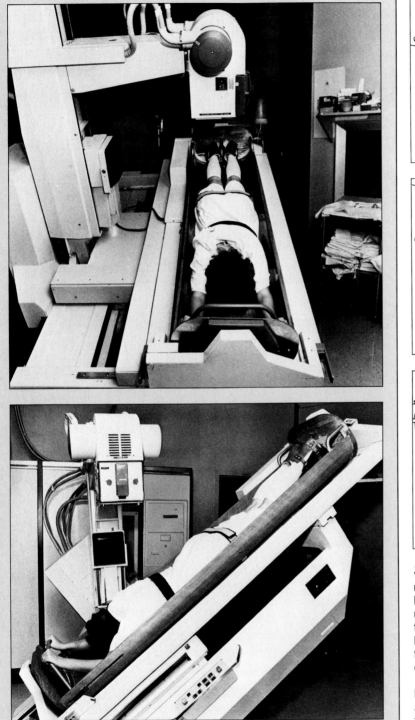

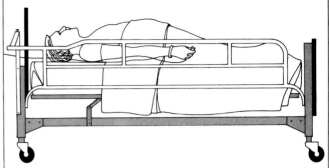

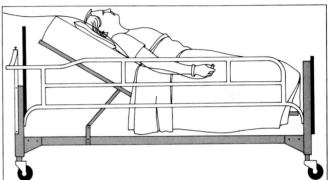

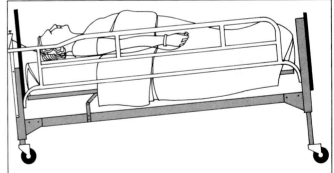

4 To study the dye flow within the subarachnoid space, the doctor will use fluoroscopy and X-rays.

To do this, the technician straps your patient into place on the myelogram table. Then, he'll move the table into seven or eight positions as he takes X-rays from each position.

5 When the X-rays are complete, Ms. Barry will be transferred to her room. Depending on the type of puncture used, and contrast agent used, she may be positioned flat, lateral, or elevated. If a positive contrast medium dye was used and then completely removed by aspiration, she will stay flat (top illustration). But if the positive contrast medium hasn't been completely removed, elevate the head of the bed to prevent dye passage into the intracranial spaces which could cause meningeal irritation (middle illustration).

If a negative contrast medium (air, gas) is used, keep her head lower than her trunk to prevent light air from rising and being trapped in the intracranial space (bottom illustration). Regardless of the contrast medium used, perform a neurocheck on Ms. Barry every 15 minutes, or as indicated. Unless she complains of nausea, encourage her to drink plenty of fluids to help replace lost CSF. Confine her to bed for 24 to 48 hours, as ordered.

Document all pre- and postprocedural care, including all patient teaching, in your nurses' notes.

Invasive tests

How pneumoencephalography works

1 *How much do you know about pneumoencephalography? If the doctor asks you to accompany your patient to the X-ray department for this procedure, would you know what to expect? If not, review these steps:*

Note: This test is usually performed in the X-ray department with a technician and doctor present.

First, the technician will position your patient in a hydraulically-controlled chair, as the photo shows.

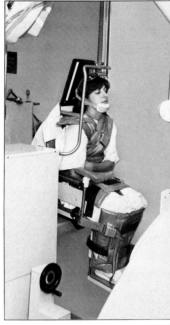

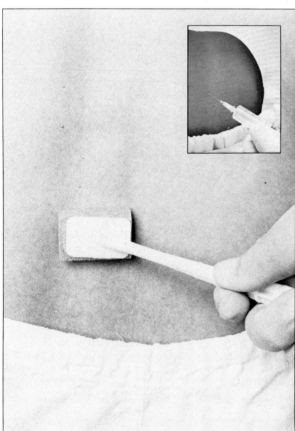

2 The doctor will prep the puncture site with povidone-iodine solution. He'll drape the area with sterile towels, leaving a 4"x4" area exposed.

[Inset] Now, the doctor will anesthetize the area.

3 The doctor inserts the lumbar puncture needle, and removes the stylet, as shown here. He'll obtain several cerebrospinal fluid (CSF) specimens (see inset). Label and send these specimens to the lab for analysis. To measure your patient's CSF pressure, he'll connect a stopcock and manometer to the spinal needle. Then he'll withdraw CSF.

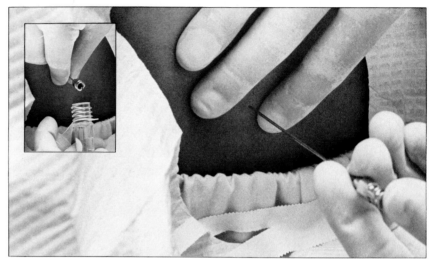

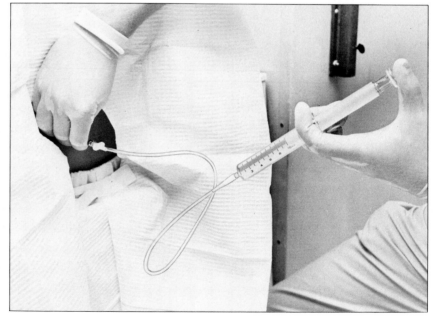

4 Next, the doctor'll inject air through the needle into your patient's subarachnoid space, and withdraw the needle. The technician will apply direct pressure to the puncture site with a gauze pad. Then, he'll cover the site with an adhesive bandage strip.

As you may know, the air injected into the patient's subarachnoid space rises and outlines the ventricular system and meninges. As the air rises, closely monitor your patient. Expect to see an increase in your patient's blood pressure, heart rate, and respiratory rate. Because the injected air increases intracranial pressure, your patient may feel light-headedness, dizziness, or may complain of headache or nausea. Keep an emesis basin and damp towel handy. Also, be sure to have emergency equipment available, such as oxygen and suction. But remember, always keep the emergency equipment out of the patient's line of vision.

5 After the air's injected, the technician will begin taking X-rays, changing the chair's position, as ordered by the doctor. He'll switch the chair into different positions, as the left-hand photos show. These position changes allow the X-ray machine to translate various views of the ventricular system and meninges onto film (see right-hand photos). Continue to reassure your patient.

When the procedure's complete, keep your patient lying flat in bed for 24 to 48 hours, as ordered. Some doctors prefer that the patient remain in a prone position after pneumoencephalography. You'll also want to elevate the patient's head as his tolerance increases.

Administer medication for headache, nausea, or vomiting, as ordered. If your patient has a continuous low-grade fever, notify the doctor. A low-grade fever may indicate a developing infection. And remember, always document everything in your nurses' notes.

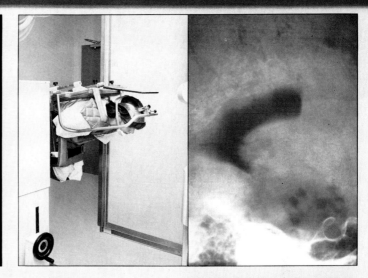

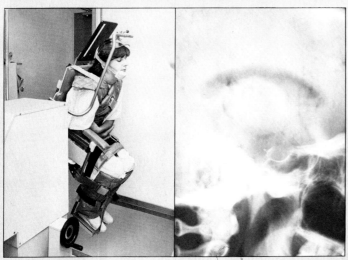

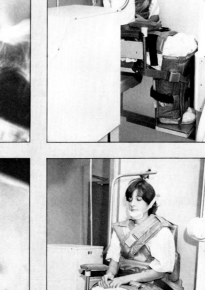

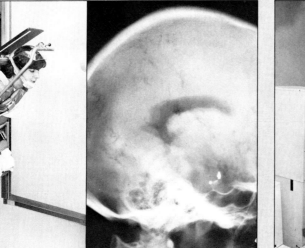

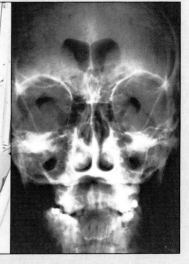

Invasive tests

Learning about brain scans

1 *Picture this: Kent McLean is scheduled for an outpatient brain scan. His doctor has ordered this test to help support a diagnosis of a left carotid artery block. Wondering how this procedure's performed? Read these guidelines:*

First, the technician instructs Mr. McLean to seat himself on a chair beneath the scintillation scanner. When he's seated, she explains the brain scan's purpose and procedure to him. She'll also have him sign a consent form.

4 Next, in place of a tourniquet, the technician wraps a blood pressure cuff around Mr. McLean's left upper arm. Before prepping the skin, she inflates the cuff slightly and looks for a suitable vein. When she finds the vein, she deflates the cuff.

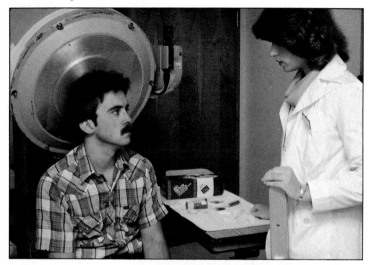

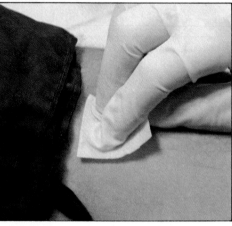

2 Now, the technician positions Mr. McLean's head against the scintillation scanner, as shown in this photo.

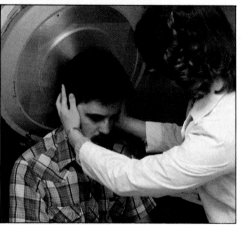

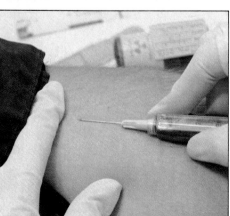

5 In this photo, the technician is prepping the puncture site with an alcohol swab. She'll let the site dry completely before inflating the cuff again.

3 To help keep Mr. McLean's head immobile during the test, the technician straps his head to the scanner. She'll adjust the strap so it's comfortable, but not too loose.

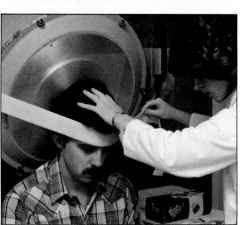

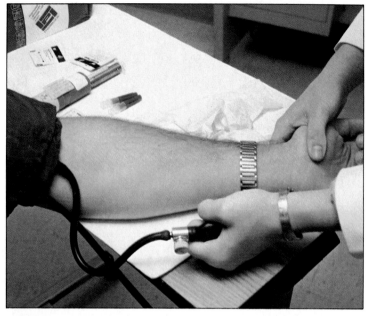

6 After inflating the cuff, the technician punctures Mr. McLean's skin with a syringe filled with a radioactive isotope medium.
Note: The syringe in this photo is prefilled with the medium.

Now, she injects the isotope.

7 As the techni-
cian removes
the syringe, she
applies direct pres-
sure to the puncture
site with a gauze
pad. Then, she
covers the site with
an adhesive ban-
dage strip.

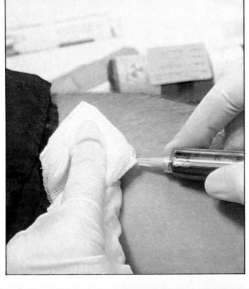

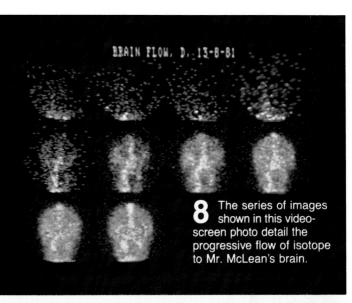

8 The series of images
shown in this video-
screen photo detail the
progressive flow of isotope
to Mr. McLean's brain.

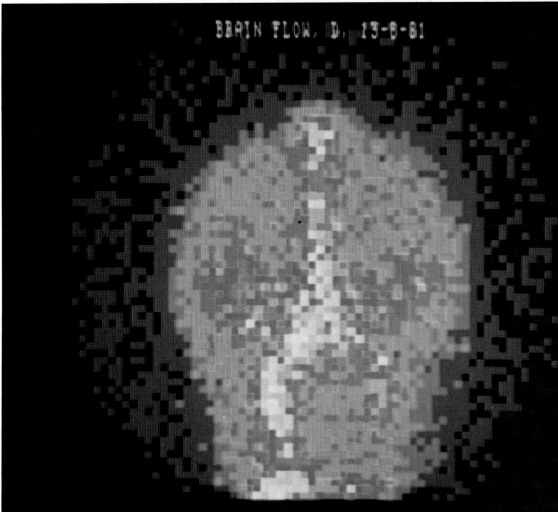

9 As you may know, the
isotope accumulates
in abnormal or damaged
brain tissue. And the
radiation emitted by the
isotope is measured
by the scintillation scanner. These measurements
are, in turn, transmitted
to the videoscreen.

Depending on the test
results, Mr. McLean will be
admitted to a unit or will
return home immediately.
Be sure to tell him that
in the next 24 hours, he'll
excrete the remaining
isotope in his urine.

Invasive tests

Understanding ventriculography

Suppose the doctor wants to relieve a patient's intracranial pressure (if lumbar and cisternal punctures are contraindicated), demonstrate ventricular system patency, locate a tumor (especially those in the posterior fossa), or detect a cerebral anomaly. He may perform ventriculography. But remember, this procedure is performed infrequently, because it can cause serious complications, such as hemorrhage from an injured blood vessel, ventriculitis from introduction of an organism, or transient blindness from damage to the optic nerves.

In most cases, ventriculography's performed in the operating room. Why? Because if a tumor's localized, a craniotomy may immediately follow the ventriculography. This possibility makes it important to prepare the patient and his family properly. Explain each step of this invasive procedure to them.

Before beginning the procedure, your patient will be seated on the operating table. Then the technician or doctor will shave his head. The doctor will inject a local anesthetic.

Next, the doctor will make an incision into the patient's scalp. Using the incision as a guide, he'll drill a hole through the bone. (Depending on the incision location, this may be either the occipital, parietal, temporal, or frontal bone.)

The doctor will pass a short, beveled needle or a small plastic tube through the opening into the lateral ventricle. Now, the doctor will inject air through the needle or tube into one of the lateral ventricles. As the air circulates through the ventricle, a series of X-rays is taken. These X-rays help the doctor with his diagnosis.

Document the procedure in your nurses' notes.

Understanding electromyography (EMG)

Anytime a patient's scheduled for EMG, you'll want to provide as much emotional support as possible. Explain the procedure to your patient and his family. Chances are, they may ask how the electromyograph works. Study the illustration below so you're better able to familiarize them with this machine.

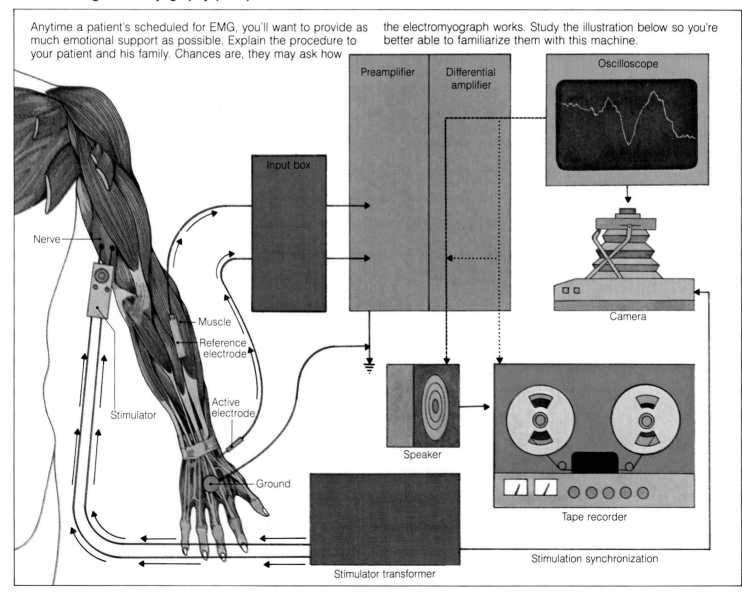

Performing electromyography (EMG)

1 *Thirty-five-year-old Fran Carrington has carpal tunnel syndrome in her left wrist. To assess the extent of peripheral nerve involvement, Ms. Carrington's doctor has ordered electromyography.* Although no special patient preparation is required for this test, you'll want to discuss EMG with Ms. Carrington. Tell her she may feel a slight tingling sensation in her arm during the test, but reassure her that the discomfort will only last a few seconds.

Now the doctor will perform this diagnostic test, following these guidelines:

First, the doctor will position Ms. Carrington on a table in the EMG area. Then, he'll explain the procedure and make sure she's signed a consent form.

2 Next, the doctor tapes a small coin-shaped plate to her left palm. This plate will serve as a ground during the test.

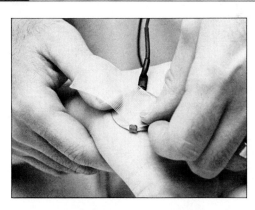

3 Now the doctor's ready to perform a nerve conduction study.

To perform this part of the test, the doctor'll tape a recording electrode over the muscle he wants to study. Then, he'll place the stimulator over the nerve to be evaluated, as shown here.

The touch of the stimulator excites a nerve in the muscle, causing an impulse to travel to the recording electrode. From here, the oscilloscope measures the electrical activity between the two points. The doctor calculates motor conduction velocity from this data.

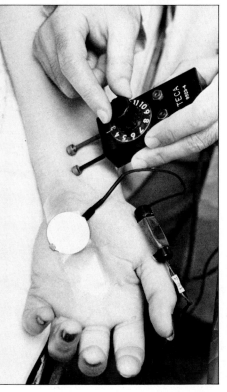

4 To assess Ms. Carrington's sensory nerves, the doctor attaches finger electrodes, as shown. As he places the stimulator over the nerve, the electrodes enable him to measure sensory action-potential.

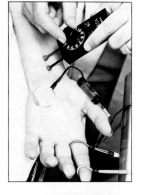

5 Now the doctor will measure Ms. Carrington's motor unit action-potential. To do this, he'll insert a small needle electrode into Ms. Carrington's muscle and study the muscle at rest. If everything's okay, a straight line will appear across the oscilloscope.

To study the muscle at minimal contraction, the doctor'll ask Ms. Carrington to extend her fingers slightly. After noting the muscle fiber pattern on the oscilloscope, he'll ask her to extend her fingers as far as possible to study maximum contraction.

By studying motor unit action-potential patterns, the doctor can identify normal or diseased muscle fibers.

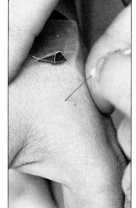

6 Here you see a readout from the oscilloscope. Following the test, Ms. Carrington can return home.

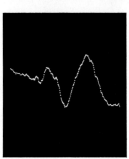

Invasive tests

Understanding cerebral angiography

Can you define cerebral angiography? You've correctly identified the term if you say it's an invasive procedure in which radiopaque dye is injected through a catheter directly or indirectly into the patient's cerebral circulatory system.

During cerebral angiography, the doctor may inject dye through a catheter directly into one or more of the patient's carotid arteries. More commonly, he may use an indirect route and inject dye through a catheter into the patient's femoral artery. In some cases, he may select the brachial or subclavian arteries.

To inject dye into the cerebral circulatory system, he'll pass a catheter through a needle into the desired artery (femoral, brachial, subclavian, or carotid). Then, he'll advance the catheter into the descending aorta, and from there into the predetermined vessel, monitoring the catheter's progress on a fluoroscope. Once the appropriate cerebral vessel is reached, the dye is injected.

Then, as the dye flows through the cerebral vasculature, a series of X-rays is taken. These X-rays help the doctor make a definitive diagnosis.

As you probably know, a cerebral angiogram defines size, location, and structural relationships of cerebral circulation abnormalities such as subdural and epidural hematomas, massive intracranial tumors, intracerebral lesions, aneurysms, and occlusive vascular diseases.

Preparing for cerebral angiography

Is your patient scheduled for cerebral angiography? If so, begin your preprocedural preparation as soon as possible. To do so, follow these steps:
• Explain the procedure to your patient and answer any questions. Reassure him that the puncture area will be locally anesthetized so he should feel only slight discomfort during the procedure.
• Make sure your patient's signed a consent form.
• Withhold foods and fluids for 6 hours prior to the procedure. Tell your patient these precautions reduce the risk of nausea or vomiting during the procedure.
• Check your patient's vital signs and perform a neurocheck routinely, or as ordered, to establish a data baseline.
• Ask the patient if he has any allergies, especially to shellfish or iodine. If he does, notify the doctor. Why? Because the dye infused during this test has an iodine base and a patient with these allergies may suffer anaphylaxis.
• Be sure a crash cart's handy. In rare cases, the dye used during the procedure may produce respiratory distress and anaphylactic shock.
• If the puncture site is located on the patient's groin or other hairy area, shave the site, according to your hospital's policy. Be sure to explain to the patient why shaving's necessary.
• Document all preprocedural teaching and preparations in your nurses' notes.

How cerebral angiography's performed

1 *How familiar are you with angiography? Would you have difficulty giving your patient a step-by-step explanation of the procedure? If so, the photos and explanations that follow will acquaint you with this procedure. Study them carefully.*

Let's say your patient, 38-year-old Kevin Nemath, a jazz pianist, arrives in the radiology department for cerebral angiography. He's been prepared properly and has signed a consent form. What's next?

First, the technician positions Mr. Nemath on a table. Then, she'll prep the groin area and drape it with sterile towels, exposing only a 4″x4″ area. After that, the doctor explains the procedure to Mr. Nemath, as shown here.

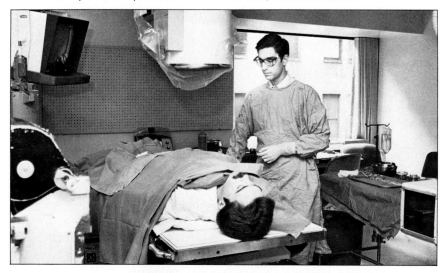

2 Now, the doctor will anesthetize the site and make a small incision over the selected artery.
Note: In this photostory, the dye will be injected into the patient's femoral artery.

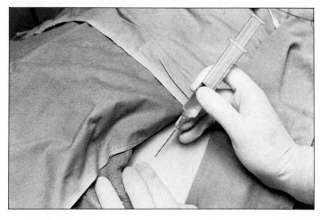

3 As shown here, the doctor inserts a hollow-bore needle (with stylet) into the incision.
After the needle enters the artery, he'll remove the stylet. When he sees blood coming from the needle, confirming correct placement, the doctor will pass a guidewire through the needle.

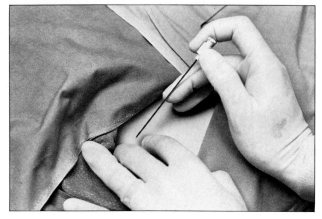

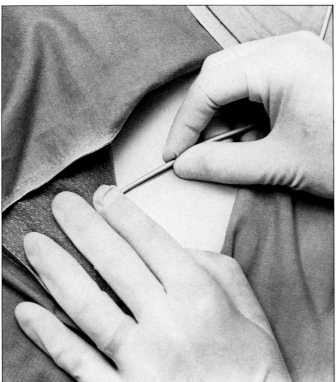

4 Checking the position of the guidewire on a fluoroscope, he'll advance the guidewire.

Then, he'll advance the catheter, as shown here, over the guidewire through the descending aorta. From there, he'll pass the catheter into the desired brain vessel, monitoring the catheter's progress on the fluoroscope.

When the catheter's in the desired blood vessel, the doctor will remove the guidewire. To prevent clot formation, he may flush the catheter with heparinized normal saline solution.

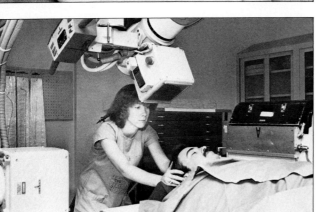

5 Next, the technician positions your patient's head under the X-ray machine, as shown in the photo. The doctor will begin injecting the contrast dye. This dye permits him to see the cerebrovascular system clearly on the fluoroscope or X-ray.

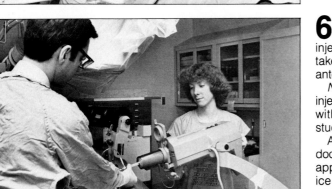

6 At this point, the doctor connects the catheter to the injector and a series of X-rays is taken rapidly from both lateral and anterior-posterior approaches.

Note: The amount of contrast dye injected and X-rays ordered varies with the blood vessels being studied.

After performing this test, the doctor will remove the catheter and apply a pressure bandage and ice pack. Then, he'll return the patient to your care.

Document the procedure in your nurses' notes.

After angiography: caring for your patient

When a patient returns to your unit after angiography, make him as comfortable as possible. Also, be sure to watch him closely for complications, using these guidelines:
• Apply ice packs to the puncture site. Doing so helps control swelling, minimizes the risk of hemorrhage, and promotes patient comfort.
• Frequently check the pressure bandage over the puncture site. Keep the bandage dry and secure.
• If bleeding occurs, apply direct pressure to the puncture site. Have a co-worker notify the doctor.
• Observe the puncture site for any redness or swelling which may indicate a hematoma. If these symptoms are present, notify the doctor.
• Take your patient's vital signs, and perform a neurocheck every 15 minutes for at least an hour, until he's stable. Then, continue to take his vital signs and perform neurochecks frequently, as ordered.
• At least once every half hour, check below the puncture site for pulse, color, warmth, and movement.
• Immobilize the patient's neck, or affected arm or leg for 4 to 6 hours to discourage bleeding. To do this, you may need sandbags.
• Make sure the patient gets at least 12 hours of complete bed rest, as ordered.
• Encourage your patient to drink plenty of fluids. Monitor his output carefully. Because contrast dye acts as a diuretic, your patient may become dehydrated.
• Follow up on test results. After the doctor has explained the results to your patient and his family, be available to answer any questions they may have.
• Document all observations in your patient's chart and in your notes. Notify the doctor of any complications immediately.

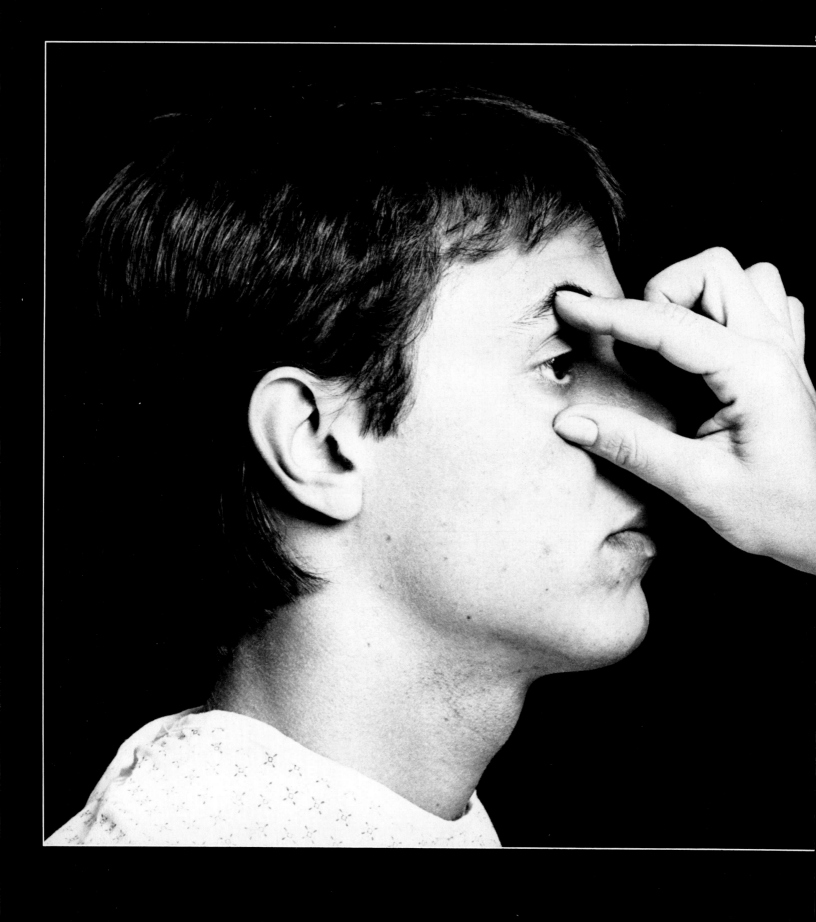

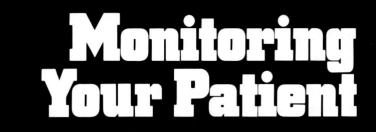

Monitoring
Your Patient

Neurocheck

Intracranial pressure

Neurocheck

As you know, a neurocheck is an ongoing evaluation of your patient's neurologic status. By comparing the information from a neurocheck with the information gathered during a thorough neurologic assessment, you can detect trends and changes in your patient's condition.

Do you know the importance of performing a neurocheck? Do you know how monitoring respiratory patterns can help you identify a change in your patient's neurologic condition? Do you know how to perform a neurocheck in an emergency situation? Can you recognize the signs of brain stem involvement?

In the following pages, we'll answer these questions and more. For example, we'll tell you how to assess a comatose patient, and what to look for when you're checking his respiratory patterns. We'll also tell you how to accurately document neurocheck findings.

To learn about neurocheck techniques, read on.

Learning about neurochecks

Has the doctor ordered an ongoing neurocheck for your patient? As you know, you'll perform this periodic assessment of your patient's neurologic system to help identify changes in his condition. But, remember, a neurocheck is designed to provide fast, frequent assessment information and is *never* a substitute for a complete neurologic assessment.

How often do you perform a neurocheck? Depending on your patient's condition and the doctor's orders, neurocheck frequency may vary from 15 minutes to 2 hours. However, in some situations, you'll perform a neurocheck more frequently; for example:
• before and after diagnostic procedures, such as a lumbar puncture or cerebral angiography
• before and after neurosurgery, such as a craniotomy
• before and after emergency intervention, such as cardiopulmonary resuscitation (CPR) or a tracheotomy
• whenever a significant change has occurred in your patient's level of consciousness.

Wondering what your patient's neurocheck will tell you? That depends on his condition. But, all neurochecks assess the following:
• *consciousness level:* may be the first indication of increasing intracranial pressure
• *motor response:* helps locate nerve weakness or damage
• *pupillary reaction (including direct response, consensual response, and size):* helps locate a space-occupying brain lesion
• *vital signs:* may identify tumor location.

As you perform neurochecks, expect to see changes in your patient's condition at different times. For example, you may see a change in his consciousness level before a change in vital signs.

When you're finished with your patient's neurocheck, be sure to document your findings clearly and accurately. Notify the doctor of any changes in your patient's condition.

Performing a neurocheck

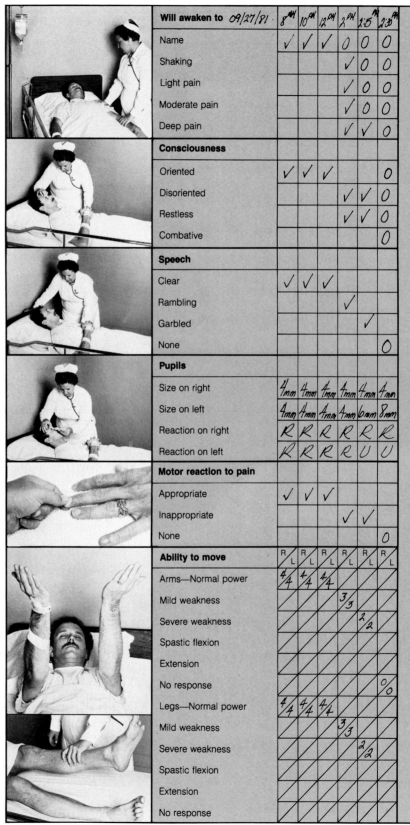

Will awaken to 09/27/81	8 AM	10 PM	12 PM	2 PM	2:15 PM	2:30 PM
Name	✓	✓	✓	0	0	0
Shaking				✓	0	0
Light pain				✓	0	0
Moderate pain				✓	0	0
Deep pain				✓	✓	0
Consciousness						
Oriented	✓	✓	✓			0
Disoriented				✓	✓	0
Restless				✓	✓	0
Combative						0
Speech						
Clear	✓	✓	✓			
Rambling				✓		
Garbled					✓	
None						0
Pupils						
Size on right	4mm	4mm	4mm	4mm	4mm	4mm
Size on left	4mm	4mm	4mm	4mm	6mm	8mm
Reaction on right	R	R	R	R	R	
Reaction on left	R	R	R	R	U	U
Motor reaction to pain						
Appropriate	✓	✓	✓			
Inappropriate				✓	✓	
None						0
Ability to move	R/L	R/L	R/L	R/L	R/L	R/L
Arms—Normal power	4/4	4/4	4/4			
Mild weakness				3/3		
Severe weakness					2/2	
Spastic flexion						
Extension						
No response						0/0
Legs—Normal power	4/4	4/4	4/4			
Mild weakness				3/3		
Severe weakness					2/2	
Spastic flexion						
Extension						
No response						

4 Normal; 3 Slight weakness; 2 Moderate weakness; 1 Minimal weakness; 0 No response; ✓ Response;
R Reactive; U Unreactive

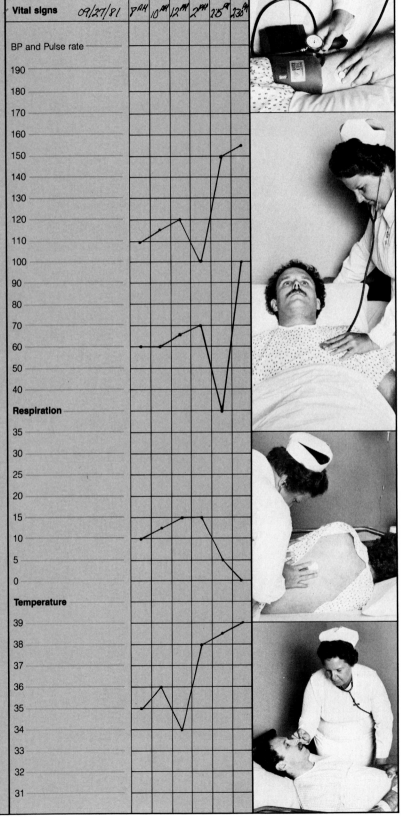

Your patient is 28-year-old Glenn Singer, who's suffered head trauma as the result of a fall. His doctor has ordered an ongoing neurocheck and it's your responsibility to initiate this procedure. Do you know how? The chart at left is an example of a neurologic check sheet you can use to document your findings. Here's how to proceed with the neurocheck.

Begin by observing Mr. Singer's level of consciousness. Is he awake, drowsy, or confused? Stuporous? Comatose? Is he alert and aware of his surroundings? Does he know where and who he is? Is he oriented to time? When you note your findings, remember to *describe* your patient's reactions.

Suppose he doesn't respond when you talk to him? Try a painful stimulus. Hold his nail between your index finger and thumb. Press his nail lightly. Consider his response normal for his condition if he pulls away.

Now, as you explain the neurocheck procedure to Mr. Singer, observe his gaze. Do both eyes work in unison? If so, consider his gaze conjugate. Carefully evaluate his pupils. Are they equal in size and shape? Accurately document their size, using a standard pupil gauge chart like the one shown on page 22.

Now you're ready to check Mr. Singer's pupillary reaction. Darken the room slightly, if possible. Tell Mr. Singer to focus on a point on the wall. Then shine your penlight into first one eye, then the other. Each pupil should constrict in response to light. To further assess pupillary reaction, you'll need to assess consensual responses. See page 21 for details.

Document the pupillary reaction as normal, sluggish, or nonreactive. But remember, nonneurologic factors, such as medication, may also affect pupillary reaction.

To check Mr. Singer's motor responses, ask him to hold both hands above his head. Have him turn his palms so they are facing the foot of the bed, and close his eyes. Can he maintain this and keep his arms steady? If Mr. Singer's one arm drifts to his side, that side may be weakened or partially paralyzed.

Test the patient's grip by asking him to squeeze your hands. Unequal pressure may indicate motor nerve or central nervous system damage.

Now ask Mr. Singer to hold up his legs, one at a time. If everything's okay, he should be able to briefly hold each leg in a raised position. If he can't, suspect motor nerve or central nervous system damage. If your patient can lift his legs, test their strength by pressing down on each leg as he attempts to lift it. Note the amount of resistance to your pressure. A weakness or inability to resist your pressure may indicate partial or complete paralysis. Notify the doctor of any changes in your patient's condition.

Next, bilaterally check your patient's blood pressure.

At this point, you'll use a stethoscope to count his apical heart rate and rhythm. Check Mr. Singer's radial, pedal, popliteal, and femoral pulses bilaterally, assessing for rate and rhythm.

Now, auscultate Mr. Singer's respirations with a stethoscope. Observe the rate and rhythm of his respirations, and document all patterns.

Notify the doctor of any changes in your patient's condition.

Finally, document all your findings on the neurocheck sheet. To do this, use a numerical scale from 4 to 0. In most hospitals, the number 4 represents a normal response.

Note: Always follow your hospital's policy when documenting your findings. And, remember to record each neurocheck.

Neurocheck

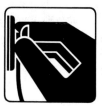

Checking vital signs

One component of a neurocheck is the ongoing assessment of your patient's vital signs. In taking these signs, you establish a data baseline. From the baseline, you'll be able to determine your patient's progress or lack of it.

Whenever you assess vital signs in a patient with a suspected neurologic disorder, ask yourself these questions:

Temperature
• Is his temperature elevated? If so, he may have an infection; for example, in the urinary tract. He may also have brain damage, especially to the hypothalamus. In addition, hyperthermia may result from a subarachnoid hemorrhage.
• Is your patient's temperature below normal? Hypothermia may indicate a brain stem lesion, overdose of a central nervous system depressant, such as a barbiturate, or insulin coma. Also, consider the possibility of overexposure to environmental elements, especially in an unconscious patient or a patient with a spinal cord injury.

Pulse
• Is your patient's pulse rapid (over 100 beats per minute) and thready? If so, he may have increasing intracranial pressure (ICP). But before you notify the doctor, be sure to rule out other possible causes of a rapid, thready pulse (tachycardia); for example, a distended bladder, shock, pain, or fever.
• Is your patient's pulse slow (under 60 beats per minute)? If so, he may be compensating for increasing ICP or have a meningeal irritation. Remember, though, a slow pulse (bradycardia) may be considered a normal sign in young or athletic patients.

Blood pressure
• Is your patient's blood pressure increasing with each neurocheck? If so, he may have increasing ICP from cerebral edema, or a subarachnoid or intracranial hemorrhage.

Respirations
• Is your patient having difficulty breathing? Are his respirations loud and moist? If so, he may have edema, pneumonia, or a developing infection. An obstructed airway may occur at anytime between or during neurochecks. Be alert for rate and quality of your patient's respirations.

Document all your findings in your nurses' notes.

Evaluating respiratory patterns in the unconscious patient

Whenever you assess an unconscious patient's vital signs, you'll also need to assess his respiratory pattern. When combined with your other assessment data, your patient's respiratory pattern can help you identify a brain lesion, as well as detail its size and location. Study the chart below to review your knowledge of respiratory patterns.

Respiratory pattern
Central neurogenic hyperventilation

Description
Sustained, regular, rapid respirations, with forced inspiration and expiration

Additional considerations
• Increased occurrence of pattern may indicate a deepening coma

Level of lesion
Midbrain or upper pons

Respiratory pattern
Apneustic breathing

Description
Prolonged inspiration, followed by inspiratory or expiratory pauses

Additional considerations
• Also known as pneumotaxic breathing or apneusis
• May be observed in certain metabolic disorders, such as hypoglycemia

Level of lesion
Pons

Respiratory pattern
Cluster breathing

Description
Irregular respirations alternating with pauses

Additional considerations
• Breathing pattern not cyclic

Level of lesion
Upper medulla or lower pons

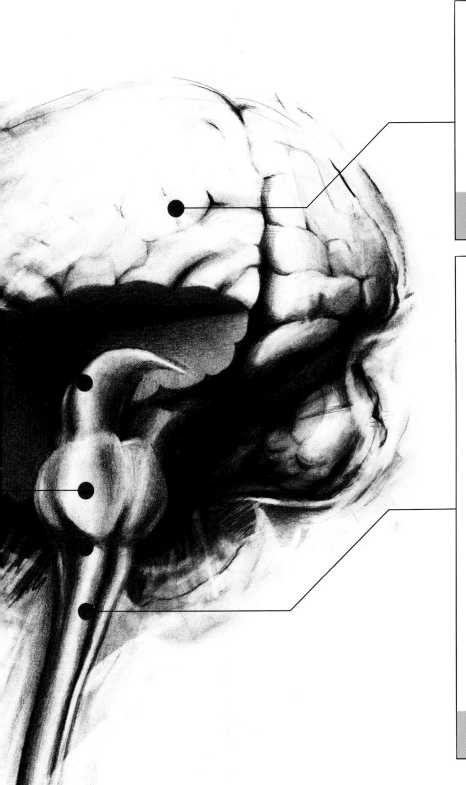

Respiratory pattern
Cheyne-Stokes

Description
Rhythmic waxing and waning of both rate and depth of respirations, alternating with brief periods of apnea

Additional considerations
• Occurs with bilateral dysfunction in cerebral hemispheres or basal ganglia area
• Pattern may also occur with some metabolic disorders such as low pH after cardiac arrest

Level of lesion
Cerebral hemispheres

Respiratory pattern
Gasping

Description
Irregular convulsive breaths accompanied by apneic periods

Respiratory pattern
Ataxic breathing

Description
Completely irregular pattern

Additional considerations
• Both ataxic and gasping patterns indicate rapidly deteriorating condition

Respiratory pattern
Depressed breathing

Description
Shallow, slow respirations

Additional considerations
• Depressed breathing is usually present in patients who have abused alcohol or drugs
• Depressed breathing may also be seen in patients who are terminally ill

Level of lesion
Medulla

Neurocheck

Understanding pupil size and reaction to light

You probably know that observing pupillary activity is an important part of a neurocheck. But do you know why? By keeping an ongoing record of your patient's pupil size and reaction to light, you may be able to recognize possible neurologic disorders and complications. Familiarize yourself with the responses and indications described below. Use this information as a guide when you assess your patient's pupillary responses.

Note: This chart describes pupil size as small and large. But, whenever you assess your patient for pupillary changes, document pupillary size by exact measurement (see page 22).

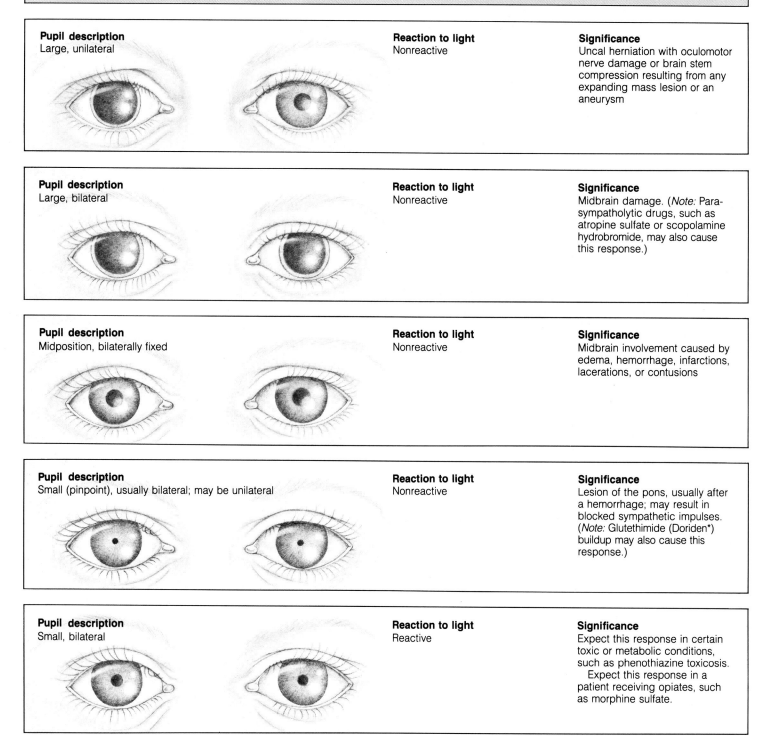

Pupil description
Large, unilateral

Reaction to light
Nonreactive

Significance
Uncal herniation with oculomotor nerve damage or brain stem compression resulting from any expanding mass lesion or an aneurysm

Pupil description
Large, bilateral

Reaction to light
Nonreactive

Significance
Midbrain damage. (*Note:* Parasympatholytic drugs, such as atropine sulfate or scopolamine hydrobromide, may also cause this response.)

Pupil description
Midposition, bilaterally fixed

Reaction to light
Nonreactive

Significance
Midbrain involvement caused by edema, hemorrhage, infarctions, lacerations, or contusions

Pupil description
Small (pinpoint), usually bilateral; may be unilateral

Reaction to light
Nonreactive

Significance
Lesion of the pons, usually after a hemorrhage; may result in blocked sympathetic impulses. (*Note:* Glutethimide (Doriden*) buildup may also cause this response.)

Pupil description
Small, bilateral

Reaction to light
Reactive

Significance
Expect this response in certain toxic or metabolic conditions, such as phenothiazine toxicosis.
Expect this response in a patient receiving opiates, such as morphine sulfate.

*Available in both the United States and in Canada

Performing an emergency neurocheck

1 *Picture this: It's your day off and you're on your way to the grocery store. At the stop sign, you spot a car smashed into a telephone pole. When you reach the car, you find the driver unconscious with her neck hyperextended against the front seat. She has a large contusion on her forehead and blood is draining from her left ear. In addition to having a head injury, you suspect she has injured her spinal cord. What should you do? Of course, you'll have to perform several assessments, including an emergency neurocheck, simultaneously. Here's how:*

First, open your patient's mouth and check her airway. Make sure it's unobstructed (see inset).

2 Check her breathing. To do this, put your ear close to her mouth and nose. You should also be able to detect air movement and see her chest and abdomen rise and fall rhythmically. If you don't see movement, place your hand on her chest.

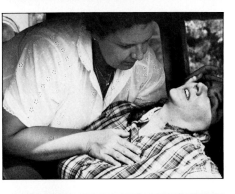

3 Next, locate her carotid artery and feel for a pulse, as shown here.

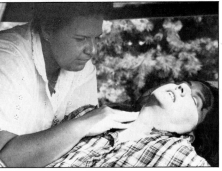

4 Then, apply direct pressure on the victim's head wound with a clean handkerchief.

Note: If you don't have a handkerchief, use any available clean cloth.

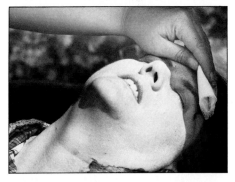

5 Now, try to assess the victim's level of consciousness. In a clear, strong voice ask, "Can you hear me?"

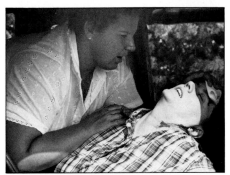

Neurocheck

Performing an emergency neurocheck continued

6 Suppose the victim does not respond to your verbal stimulation. Then, squeeze her nail. Does she respond to painful stimuli? Note your findings.

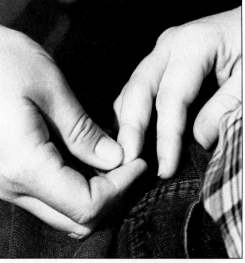

7 Inspect the victim's pupils. To do this, lift both eyelids at the same time, as shown in this photo. Are her pupils equal in size? Do they respond similarly to light? Do her eyes wander?

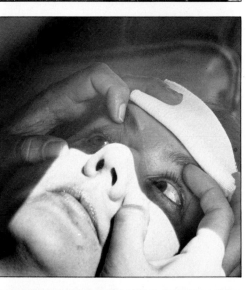

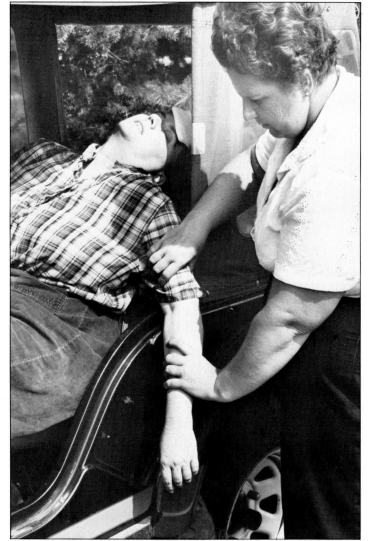

8 Without moving the victim's head, look for any cuts or bruises. Also check her nose, mouth, and ears. Observe for blood or clear fluid drainage. Draining blood or cerebrospinal fluid may indicate a skull fracture.

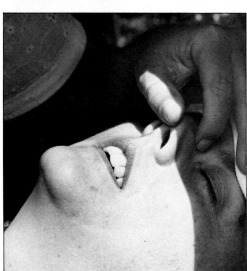

9 Next, check the victim's arms, legs, and abdomen for signs of injury (see above). Also look for possible fractures.
As you wait for other health care professionals to arrive, routinely reassess the victim's airway, respiratory rate, and pulse (as shown at right). Pay attention to the victim's breathing, so you can describe it later. For example, does the victim suddenly take a deep breath, hold it, and exhale? This is called an apneustic pattern and may indicate brain stem involvement.

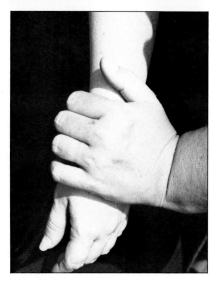

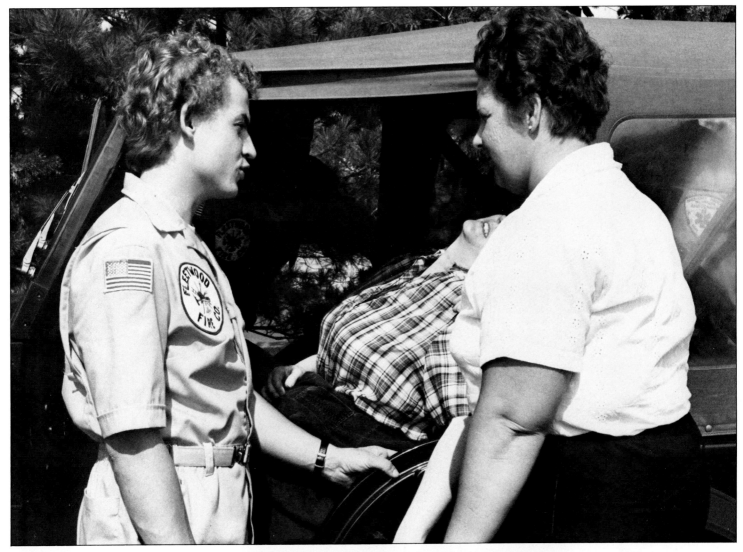

10 When the ambulance crew arrives, advise them of your observations, as the nurse is doing here.

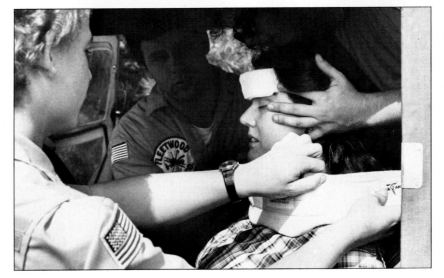

11 Now as one ambulance attendant applies head traction, the other attendant will apply a cervical collar to the victim's neck. After the collar's in place, the attendant will continue to support the victim's head and neck until her head is stabilized on a short spine board.

Neurocheck

Performing an emergency neurocheck continued

12 To safely remove a victim with a suspected spinal cord injury from a car, the ambulance personnel will apply a short spine board (left photo).

Important: Never allow a victim with suspected spinal cord injury to be moved without being immobilized using a cervical collar and spine board.

Before securing the victim to the short spine board, the attendants support the head and neck with folded towels (middle photo).

Now, the attendant secures the straps on the spine board (right photo).

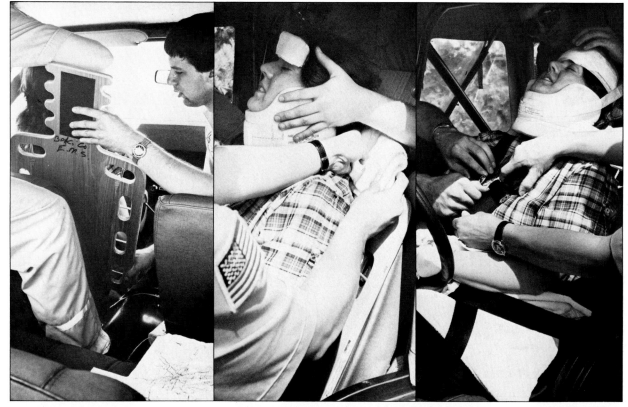

13 Next, the ambulance attendants transfer the victim to a long spine board.

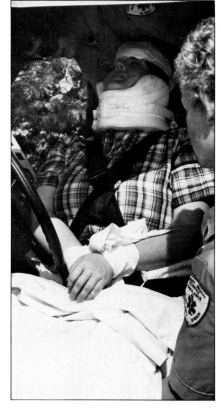

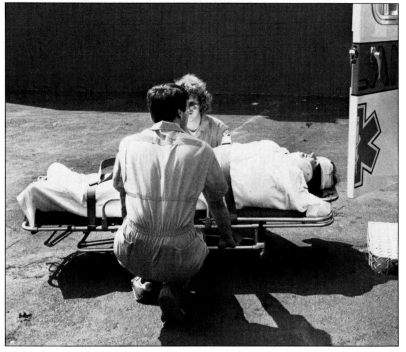

14 The ambulance attendants transfer the victim on the long board onto the litter. In this photo, she's being moved into the ambulance. On the way to the hospital, the attendants will continue to perform ongoing neurochecks.

Identifying brain stem involvement

1 *Consider this possibility: Sara Bangor, a 32-year-old homemaker, was admitted to your unit at 4 p.m. after suffering intractable headaches. At that time, the doctor ordered a neurocheck every 30 minutes. Now, 4 hours later, you note a rapid decline in Ms. Bangor's consciousness level. To help confirm your suspicions, perform these additional tests.*

First, hold Ms. Bangor's eyelids open. If her eyes appear fixed straight ahead, quickly—but gently—turn her head to the right. If everything's okay, her eyes will appear to move conjugately toward the center of her body (left of her eye socket). But if Ms. Bangor's eyes remain stationary in the center, or to the right of her eye sockets, her doll's eye reflex is absent indicating a deteriorating consciousness level. Notify the doctor immediately.

2 Now, squeeze her thumbnail with your thumb and index finger. If all's well for a patient in her condition, she'll pull away from the painful stimulus.

Suppose she draws up her arms in full flexion on her chest and extends her legs stiffly, as shown here. This is called decorticate posturing and is a sign of brain stem damage.

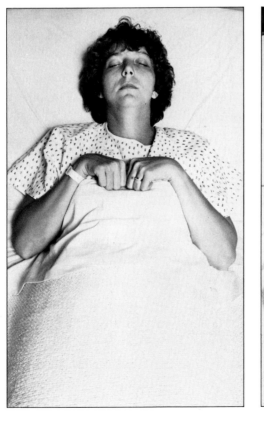

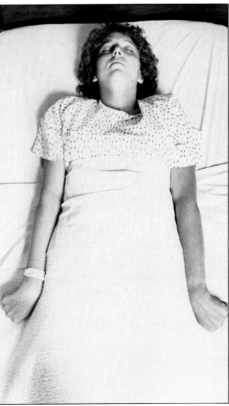

3 What if after squeezing Ms. Bangor's thumbnail, she extends her arms and legs stiffly with her palms turned outward? This action is called decerebrate posturing and usually indicates extensive brain stem damage.

If she doesn't respond to painful stimulus, consider her brain stem damage ominous.

Document your findings in your nurses' notes.

Neurocheck

Neurocheck sheet: some guidelines

Whenever or wherever you perform a neurocheck, your observations and thorough documentation may save a patient's life. So, while performing a neurocheck on your patient, keep these important points in mind:

• Be specific and complete when you describe your observations. Document clearly.

☎ *Nursing tip:* At the end of your shift, ask a co-worker from the next shift to assist you with a neurocheck. Doing so helps to ensure neurocheck continuity.

• Be complete. Perform a neurocheck as often as ordered. Missing even one may mean missing a critical sign about your patient's changing condition.

• Monitor all patients as if they have a serious neurologic disorder until tests and repeated neurochecks prove otherwise.

Using a computer-guided neurologic assessment

Does the neurologic assessment sheet at right look strange to you? If you're like most nurses, it probably does. This printout is the result of a computer-guided neurologic assessment. Some hospitals have found this system useful in providing fast, accurate, and objective interpretations of neurocheck data.

Wondering how a computer-guided assessment works? First, you'll perform a neurocheck on your patient. Then, instead of documenting your finding on a neurologic check sheet, you'll document your findings on a multiple choice questionnaire. At this point, you (or a data processor) will enter the information from the questionnaire into the computer. From there, the computer organizes your clinical findings into a meaningful printout.

Sound easy? It is, but the computer-guided program has some disadvantages. For starters, the program is expensive and requires special staff training. And remember, the accuracy of the computer printout depends on your ability to accurately assess your patient and interpret your findings.

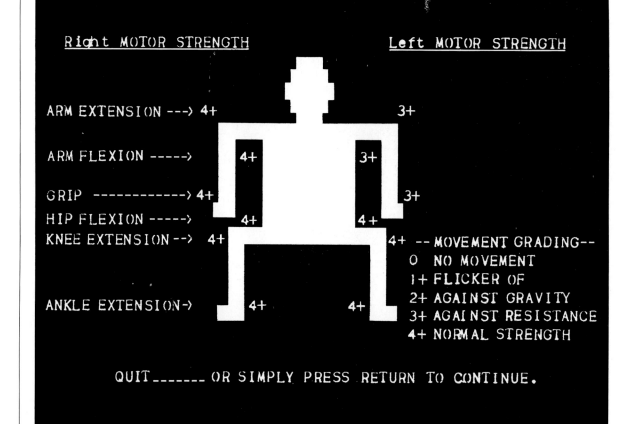

Intracranial pressure

Let's imagine you're caring for a patient with a massive brain lesion. The doctor orders intracranial pressure (ICP) monitoring. Do you know how to help prepare your patient for ICP monitoring? Do you know how to identify a C wave when reading an ICP waveform? Can you interpret it?

There are three invasive ICP monitoring systems. Are you aware of the advantages and disadvantages of each? Do you know how to observe signs of rising ICP? Can you change your patient's head dressing?

Read the following pages for answers to these questions. We've included valuable charts, illustrations, and photos to familiarize you with ICP monitoring equipment.

Learning about intracranial pressure (ICP)

As you probably remember from the first section, the skull provides a hard, inflexible casing for the brain. It protects the brain from injury and infection. Now, keep in mind that within the skull, a delicate balance exists between brain tissue, blood and cerebrospinal fluid (CSF). In some cases, such as disease or severe trauma, the balance between these brain components becomes upset. When one of these components significantly increases in volume, the remaining components must proportionately decrease in volume. If they don't, intracranial pressure (ICP) within the skull will *rise* quickly and dangerously (simulated at right).

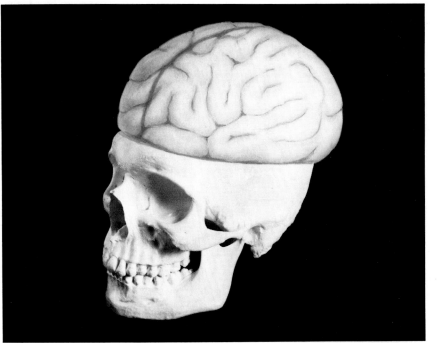

Wonder what happens when ICP rises? For starters, the increased pressure prevents blood from perfusing the brain's cerebral cortex. This deprives the brain of its blood and oxygen supply. As you may know, adequate perfusion depends on a cerebral perfusion pressure (CPP) of 60 to 90 mm Hg.

Usually, a patient undergoing ICP monitoring is also undergoing continuous arterial blood pressure monitoring. So how do you calculate CPP? It's simple. Subtract the patient's ICP from his mean systemic arterial pressure (MSAP). To do this, use this formula: MSAP - ICP = CPP.

Of course, the brain accounts for approximately 85% of the skull's contents. So in most cases, the brain compensates for increasing

ICP by regulating the volume of blood and CSF with one of these techniques:
• *Pressure autoregulation*. Cerebral blood flow must remain stable, regardless of fluctuation in MSAP. So, if MSAP rises, the cerebral blood vessels constrict, limiting blood flow to the head. And, if MSAP falls, cerebral blood vessels dilate.
• *Metabolic autoregulation*. Receptors in the brain constantly analyze blood gases. If the level of wastes (CO_2 and lactic acid) rises, the cerebral blood vessels dilate and increase the flow of oxygenated blood. Conversely, if the receptors detect a high oxygen level in the blood, the cerebral blood vessels constrict and limit the flow of oxygenated blood.
• *CSF regulation*. If ICP rises, CSF can be displaced into the spinal canal through several openings, primarily

the foramen of Luschka and the foramen of Magendie. The dura mater that covers the spinal canal is loosely attached and readily expands to allow departing CSF. At the same time, the arachnoid villi will increase their absorption of CSF into the venous sinuses.

But what happens when the brain can no longer compensate for a small volume increase? This inability to compensate is called decompensation, a life-threatening cycle that demands immediate attention.

Why is it serious? During decompensation, the patient's cerebral blood flow is controlled by the systemic arterial pressure (SAP) alone. If SAP should rise during decompensation, the following cyclic adjustments occur: When cerebral blood perfusion becomes inadequate and the brain's blood supply becomes dimin-

ished, then the ICP increases, causing CPP to decrease. As a result, serum O_2 levels decrease and CO_2 and lactic acid levels increase. Now, the cerebral vessels dilate and the additional blood flow increases the ICP again, starting the same cycle.

How can the doctor evaluate decompensation? If the patient has a ventricular catheter in place, the doctor may perform a volume-pressure response test. To do this, he'll inject a small amount of sterile I.V. saline solution into the ventricular catheter. Then, he'll watch the monitor to determine if the patient's ICP rises sharply in response to this sudden increase in intraventricular volume. If it does, the doctor will be likely to order immediate therapy to lower the patient's ICP. (To learn about different types of ICP therapy, read the information on pages 82 to 83.)

Intracranial pressure

Intracranial pressure (ICP) monitoring: some indications

Does your patient need ICP monitoring? He may, if he has any of the following conditions:
- massive brain lesion
- head trauma with bleeding and edema
- overproduction and/or insufficient cerebrospinal fluid absorption, causing hydrocephalus
- congenital hydrocephalus
- cerebral hemorrhage
- encephalitis, particularly Reye's syndrome.

Also, suspect the need for ICP monitoring if you note signs of increased ICP pressure, such as:
- headache or vomiting
- deteriorating respiratory pattern
- deteriorating consciousness level
- deteriorating motor function.

Be sure to notify the doctor of any of these signs. He may decide to order ICP monitoring for your patient.

But remember, ICP monitoring is a supplement, not a substitute for observing your patient. In most cases, an ICP monitoring device will warn of rising ICP. But that doesn't reduce the need to carefully watch your patient's clinical signs. As you watch the monitor, continue to perform neurochecks, and document your findings.

Preparing your patient for intracranial monitoring

Let's consider the case of Winifred Tolland, a 67-year-old retired garment worker. After suffering severe head trauma from an automobile accident 2 weeks ago, her family felt confident she would be released from the hospital any day. Now, her level of consciousness has deteriorated and she's scheduled for ICP monitoring using a subarachnoid screw. The doctor explained the purpose, equipment, and procedure to her family, but they were too upset to ask any questions. How can you help?

As you know, preparing Ms. Tolland and her family emotionally for this procedure is a major part of your nursing responsibility. When you speak with her family, bring along illustrations of ICP pressure monitoring systems.

Clearly explain to the patient and her family that the doctor will make a small hole in her skull and insert the monitoring device. Then, he'll connect the monitor to the machine. Tell them the monitor will enable the doctor to identify what is happening in Ms. Tolland's brain, and alert him to any changes.

Assure the family that the procedure will not affect brain tissue or functioning. And remind them that following removal of the catheter or screw, the puncture site will heal with routine nursing care.

Nurses' guide to intracranial pressure (ICP) monitoring systems

How familiar are you with ICP monitoring systems? For example, do you know the difference between a ventricular catheter and a subarachnoid screw? If your patient has an epidural sensor, do you know how to check the sensor before using it?

The chart at right answers these questions and gives you specific information on the three most commonly used ICP monitoring devices. In addition, remember these general guidelines when setting up an ICP monitoring system:

Note: Procedures vary from hospital to hospital. Always follow your hospital's policy.
- Maintain strict aseptic technique throughout. Do everything possible to reduce the risk of infection.
- Keep all stopcock ports capped, unless you must open one to expel air or balance the transducer. Before you begin setting up, replace any open stopcock caps with closed ones.
- Expel air from the tubing and stopcock ports before connecting the line to the patient. Air in the line will damp the waveform, giving an inaccurate ICP reading.
- Never flush any fluid into the patient's cranial cavity. Doing so will raise his already elevated ICP and may also cause infection.

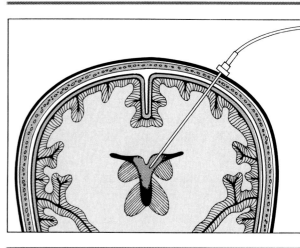

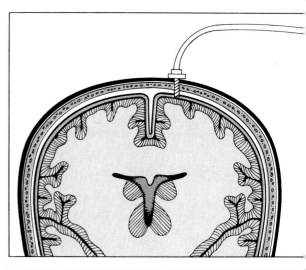

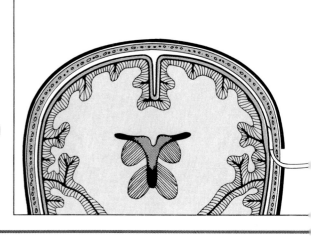

Monitoring system	Use	Nursing considerations
Ventricular catheter Cannula and reservoir inserted into the brain's ventricle through a twist-drill hole in the skull.	• To measure ICP • To evaluate volume-pressure responses • To drain large amount of cerebrospinal fluid (CSF) • To instill contrast medium	• Expect catheter placement to be difficult if ventricle's collapsed, swollen, or displaced. • Monitor patient closely for infections, such as meningitis and ventriculitis. Remember, this monitor is the most invasive of the three systems. • Check catheter patency frequently. If catheter becomes occluded with blood or brain tissue, notify the doctor. He may flush it with a small amount of sterile I.V. saline solution. • Be sure stopcocks are positioned properly. Incorrect stopcock placement may create excessive CSF drainage, causing a sudden drop in ICP and possible brain herniation. • Note any sudden changes in ICP reading. A collapsed ventricle may compress the catheter, causing a false reading. • Recalibrate transducer and monitor frequently.
Subarachnoid screw Steel screw with a sensor tip inserted through a twist-drill hole in skull. Small incision made in the dura mater allows screw and tip to connect with subarachnoid space. Transducer attached to screw converts CSF pressure to electrical impulses.	• To measure ICP • To provide access for CSF sampling	• Monitor patient closely for signs of infection. • Recalibrate the transducer and monitor frequently. • Check screw patency frequently. If screw becomes occluded with blood or brain tissue, notify the doctor. He may flush it with a small amount of sterile I.V. saline solution.
Epidural sensor Tiny fiber-optic sensor inserted in brain's epidural space through burr hole in skull. Sensor cable plugs directly into monitor. Because this system cannot be recalibrated when affected by heat or pressure, its reliability remains controversial.	• To measure ICP	• Monitor patient closely for signs of infection. But remember, this monitor is the least invasive of the three systems. • Check sensor's accuracy before each use. To do this, set the monitor on MANUAL TEST and apply a known pressure. If the readings aren't identical, discard the sensor. Obtain a new one and repeat the test. • Be sure sensor's plugged tightly into monitor.

Intracranial pressure

Applying a head bandage

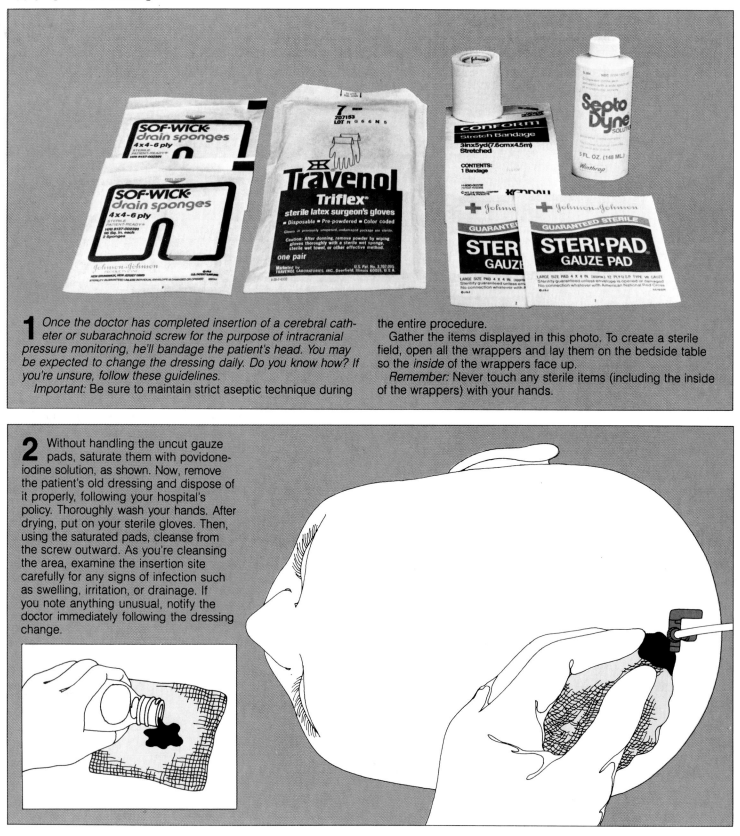

1 Once the doctor has completed insertion of a cerebral catheter or subarachnoid screw for the purpose of intracranial pressure monitoring, he'll bandage the patient's head. You may be expected to change the dressing daily. Do you know how? If you're unsure, follow these guidelines.

Important: Be sure to maintain strict aseptic technique during the entire procedure.

Gather the items displayed in this photo. To create a sterile field, open all the wrappers and lay them on the bedside table so the *inside* of the wrappers face up.

Remember: Never touch any sterile items (including the inside of the wrappers) with your hands.

2 Without handling the uncut gauze pads, saturate them with povidone-iodine solution, as shown. Now, remove the patient's old dressing and dispose of it properly, following your hospital's policy. Thoroughly wash your hands. After drying, put on your sterile gloves. Then, using the saturated pads, cleanse from the screw outward. As you're cleansing the area, examine the insertion site carefully for any signs of infection such as swelling, irritation, or drainage. If you note anything unusual, notify the doctor immediately following the dressing change.

3 Now, place the two precut drain sponges around the screw or catheter, as shown here. Be sure that their edges overlap completely.

Note: Keep the screw or catheter exposed and easily accessible.

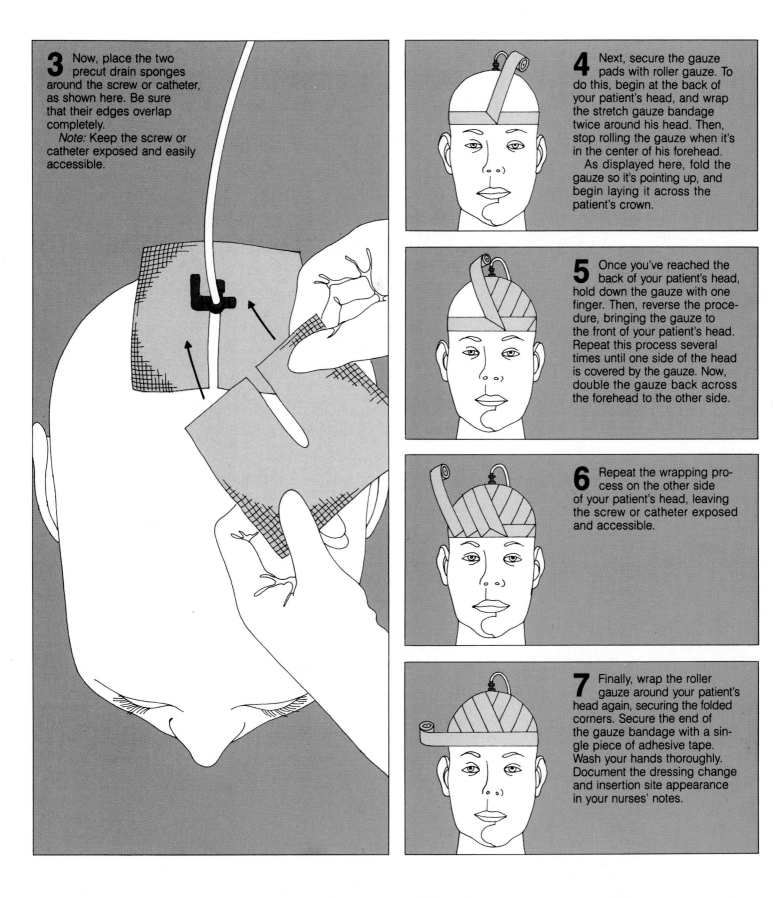

4 Next, secure the gauze pads with roller gauze. To do this, begin at the back of your patient's head, and wrap the stretch gauze bandage twice around his head. Then, stop rolling the gauze when it's in the center of his forehead.

As displayed here, fold the gauze so it's pointing up, and begin laying it across the patient's crown.

5 Once you've reached the back of your patient's head, hold down the gauze with one finger. Then, reverse the procedure, bringing the gauze to the front of your patient's head. Repeat this process several times until one side of the head is covered by the gauze. Now, double the gauze back across the forehead to the other side.

6 Repeat the wrapping process on the other side of your patient's head, leaving the screw or catheter exposed and accessible.

7 Finally, wrap the roller gauze around your patient's head again, securing the folded corners. Secure the end of the gauze bandage with a single piece of adhesive tape. Wash your hands thoroughly. Document the dressing change and insertion site appearance in your nurses' notes.

Intracranial pressure

What to do when your patient has elevated intracranial pressure (ICP)

Your patient, Bill Curley, suffered a gunshot wound to his head. As you probably know, Mr. Curley needs treatment for increased ICP. The doctor will probably select one of the treatments below.

Study this chart carefully to find out how each treatment works, and how you can help.

Treatment	Purpose	Nursing considerations
Administration of osmotic diuretics, for example, mannitol (Osmitrol*) by I.V. drip or bolus	• Reduces cerebral edema, decreasing intracranial contents	• Monitor fluids and electrolytes (including osmolarity) closely. Treatment may cause rapid dehydration. • Watch for a rebound rise in ICP from treatment. • Avoid storing mannitol at low temperatures, as it may crystallize.
Administration of steroids I.V.; for example, dexamethasone (Decadron*)	• Reduces cerebral edema by lowering sodium and water concentration in the brain	• Give steroid with antacids orally and cimetidine (Tagamet*) orally or I.V., as ordered, to prevent peptic ulcers. • Watch for signs and symptoms of gastrointestinal bleeding, such as dark-colored stools, low blood pressure, dizziness, nausea, and vomiting large amounts of bright red blood.
Withdrawal of cerebrospinal fluid (CSF) by performing a lumbar or cisternal puncture, or using a ventricular catheter	• Reduces CSF volume	• If the doctor performs a lumbar or cisternal puncture, perform a neurocheck frequently after the procedure. Remember, a sudden drop in ICP may allow brain herniation. • If the doctor uses a ventricular catheter, prevent sepsis by changing the tubing and drainage bag using strict aseptic technique.
Restriction of fluid	• Reduces cerebral edema and decreases brain volume, provided the brain's not diseased	• Monitor fluids and electrolytes (including osmolarity) closely. Dehydration below 325 Osm may have little therapeutic value. • Maintain fluid restrictions according to the doctor's orders. (He'll probably restrict an adult patient to 1200 or 1500 ml/day.) • Document the patient's fluid intake and output accurately. Remember to include all I.V. medications in your calculations.
Hyperventilation with hand-held resuscitator	• Helps blow off CO_2 which causes constriction of blood vessels and reduction of cerebral blood flow	• Monitor arterial blood gas (ABG) measurement. Notify the doctor if CO_2 continues to rise. He may want to increase the rate of ventilations.
Administration of barbiturates to induce coma; for example, phenobarbitol (Luminal*)	• Decreases cerebral metabolic rate; decreases cerebral blood flow	• Monitor vital signs regularly, especially respirations. • Give barbiturates, as ordered. Remember, when performing neurochecks on your patient, you'll have difficulty assessing his mental status when he's receiving barbiturates.
Surgical removal of skull bone flap	• Allows for expansion of cranial contents	• Keep site clean and dry to prevent infection. • Maintain strict aseptic technique when redressing the site.

*Available in both the United States and in Canada

Intracranial pressure (ICP) waveforms: What do they indicate?

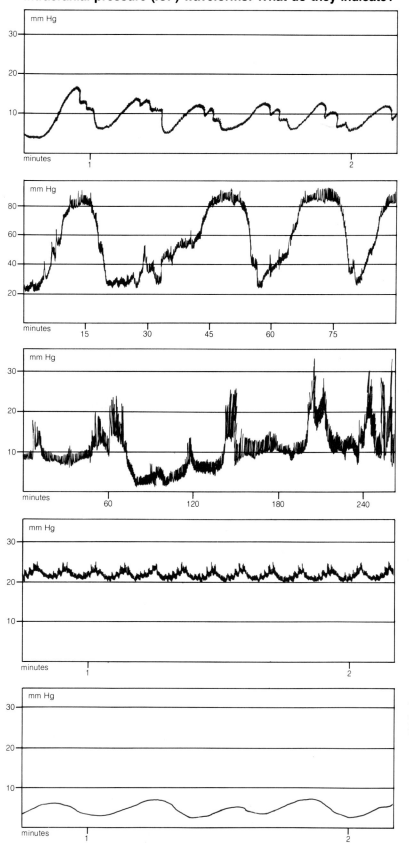

1 *Remember Winifred Tolland? Now she's receiving ICP monitoring. Do you know how to interpret the waveforms accurately? Keep in mind you'll have to study a series of readings to accurately assess her ICP and progress. The following information will tell you how. Read it carefully.*

The illustration at left shows a normal ICP waveform. Note the steep upward systolic slope followed by the downward diastolic slope with dicrotic notch. In most cases, this waveform occurs continuously, and indicates an ICP measurement between 4 and 15 mm Hg. As you know, your patient's normal pattern should be within this range.

2 The most clinically significant ICP waveforms are A waves (sometimes called plateau waves), shown here. The A waves may reach elevations of 50 to 100 mm Hg—and then drop sharply. They may come and go, spiking with temporary rises in thoracic pressure. As you probably know, activities such as sustained coughing or straining with bowel movements may cause a temporary rise in thoracic pressure.

But if A waves recur, or if they're sustained for several minutes, notify the doctor immediately. Recurring A waves indicate a rapid, dangerous rise in ICP and a reduced ability to compensate. Sustained A waves may also indicate irreversible brain damage.

3 B waves appear sharp and rhythmic, with a sawtooth pattern. They occur every 1½ to 2 minutes and may reach elevations of 50 mm Hg. These high elevations are not sustained, however. The clinical significance of B waves isn't clear, but they seem to occur more frequently with decreasing compensation. Sometimes B waves precede A waves. Watch them closely. If you see this pattern appearing with frequency, notify the doctor.

4 As you can see, C waves are rapid and rhythmic, and appear less sharp than B waves. They may fluctuate with respiration or systemic blood pressure changes. Keep in mind, though, that C waves are not clinically significant.

5 This illustration shows a damped waveform. This waveform usually signals a problem with the line or transducer. If you see this waveform, check to see if the line's obstructed or the transducer needs rebalancing.

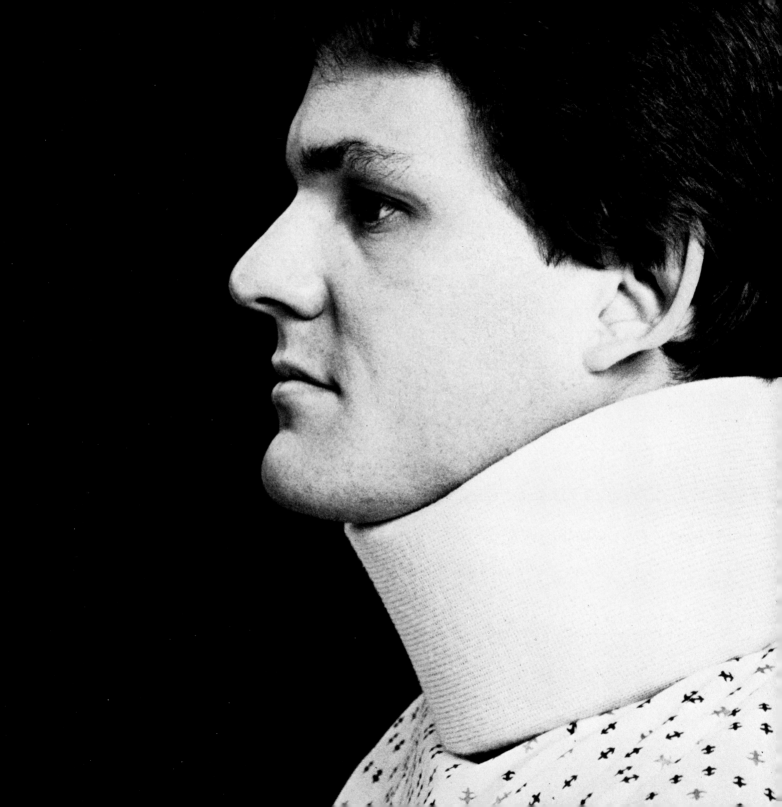

Dealing with Neurologic Problems

Diseases and disorders

Nursing care

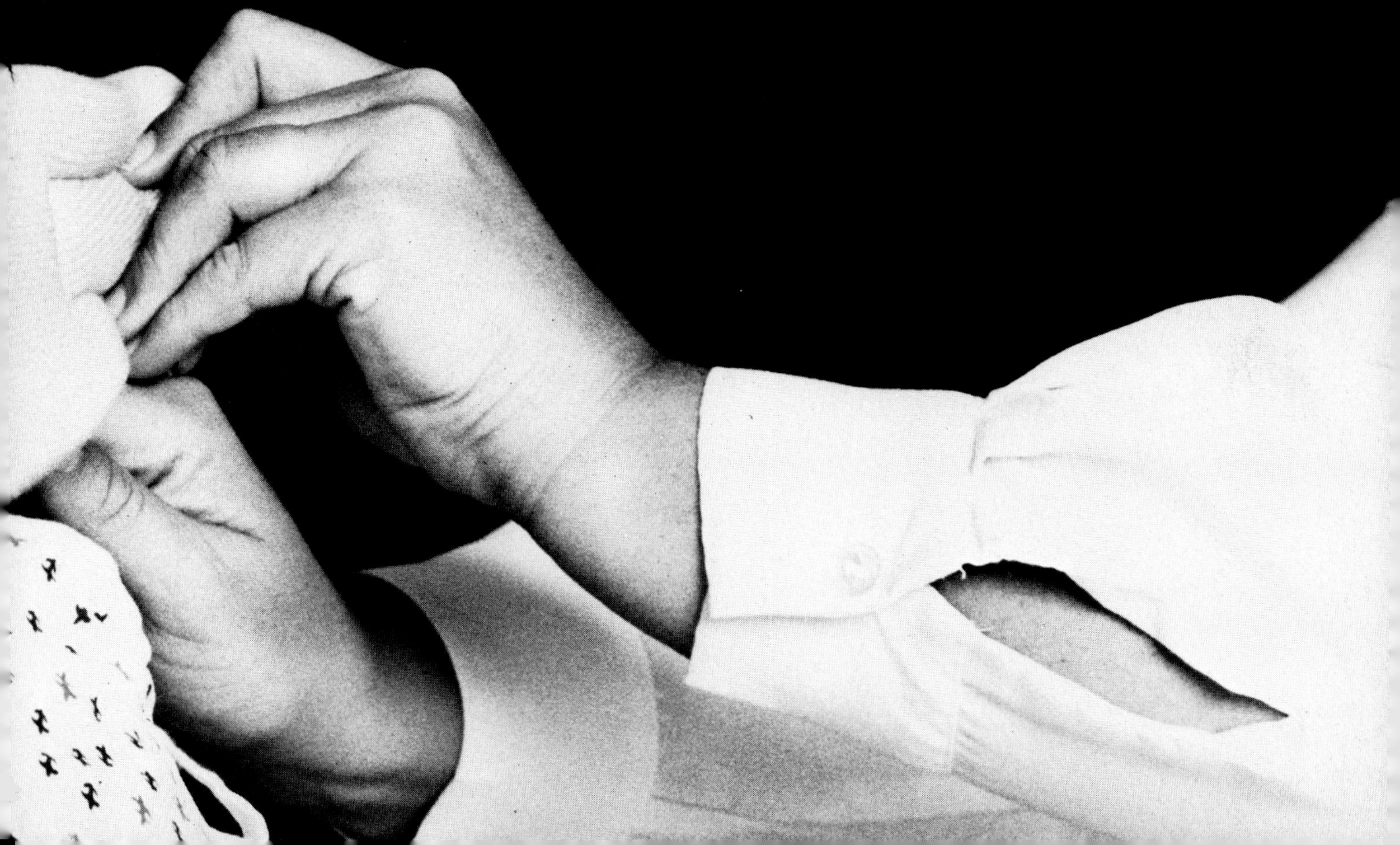

Diseases and disorders

What is a neurologic disorder? It may be any one of the following:
• traumatic injury to the brain, brain stem, spinal cord, or peripheral nervous system; for example, a concussion or contusion
• associated injury to surrounding structures; for example, a skull or facial fracture
• nontraumatic injury affecting the brain, spinal cord, and nerves; for example, a tumor or aneurysm
• secondary injury and complications; for example, a hematoma or infection.

In the pages that follow, we're going to explore common traumatic and nontraumatic neurologic injuries, so you'll know what to expect, know what to look for, and know what immediate action you can take.

Nurses' guide to traumatic neurologic injuries

Whenever you care for a patient with a traumatic head injury, suspect possible associated skull and facial fractures. Be prepared to provide treatment for these injuries, as well. In some cases, you'll be able to confirm a facial or skull fracture by observing deformities. In other cases, your patient may need an X-ray to confirm a fracture.

The chart below will acquaint you with some common types of traumatic neurologic injuries. We've illustrated each injury to make differentiation easier.

Contusion (A bruising of the brain)
Cause: A blow to the head bruises the brain directly, such as when a person is hit forcefully on the head. Such a blow drives the brain into the opposite side of the skull, which causes more bruising (contrecoup injury). Or, a person's head may be hurled forward, such as in a car accident, causing the brain to slap against the back of the skull. Then the head is stopped abruptly, causing the brain to slap against the front of the skull (acceleration-deceleration injury).
Signs and symptoms: Alteration in vital signs (respirations: normal, ataxic, periodic, or very rapid; temperature: high, accompanied by diaphoresis; pulse: rapid); pupils are usually small, equal, and reactive; loss of normal eye movement; unilateral paralysis or, if severe, total limb paralysis; decerebrate or decorticate posturing; and loss of consciousness.

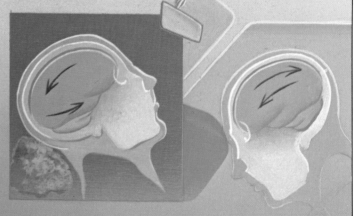

Concussion (Functional impairment of the brain)
Cause: A blow to the head or face, such as when a person hits his head on a door.
Signs and symptoms: Disorientation to person, time, and place; physical restlessness or combativeness; blurred or double vision; brief unconsciousness; verbal abusiveness; large pupils; dizziness; headache; and amnesia.

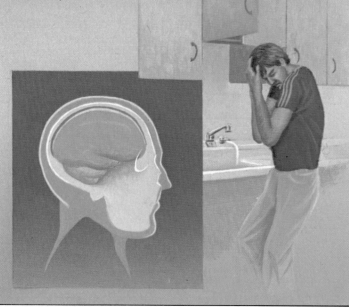

Penetrating skull injury (Presence of a foreign object in the brain)
Cause: An object, such as a knife, passes through the skull and lodges in the brain.
Signs and symptoms: Open wound with an observable object (such as a knife or an ice pick) protruding from the head; loss of normal eye movement; loss of consciousness; restlessness; irritability; bleeding; and headache.

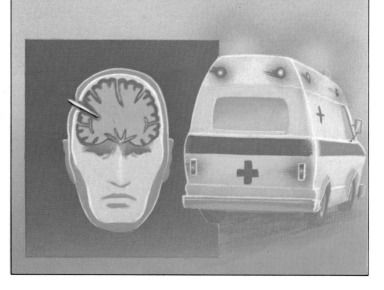

Lacerations (Penetration of skull and brain)
Cause: A blow, such as from a hammer, that fractures the skull and lacerates the brain. In other cases, it may be caused by the entrance of an object, such as a bullet, that passes through skull and brain but doesn't lodge there.
Signs and symptoms: Observable wound at entrance and exit; loss of consciousness; and bleeding.

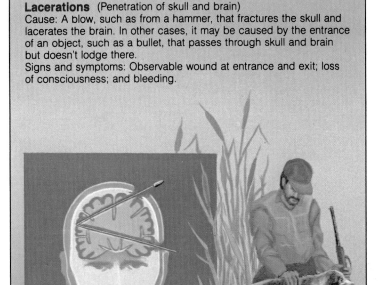

Spinal hyperextension (Extreme stretching of the spinal cord against the ligamenta flava)
Cause: Direct or indirect violence, such as a fall in which the person lands on his jaw, causing the head to bend back sharply. This, in turn, may cause contusion of the dorsal columns and posterior dislocation of the vertebrae.
Signs and symptoms: Central cervical cord injury syndrome (more motor loss in arms than in legs, varying degrees of sensory loss and bladder dysfunction); neck and back pain, which may radiate; obvious spinal deformity; decreased sensory levels; limited body movements; and unconsciousness.

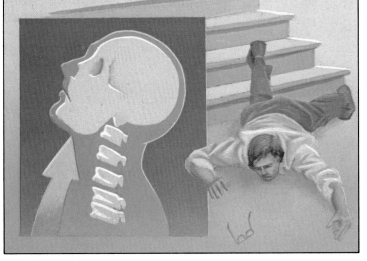

Spinal hyperflexion (Extreme movement of a portion of the spinal column beyond its normal range of motion)
Cause: Direct or indirect violence, such as a car accident in which the person strikes the steering wheel, creating a wedging force on the spinal vertebrae. This force often crushes the vertebrae, driving bony fragments posteriorly into the spinal canal.
Signs and symptoms: Spinal shock syndrome (complete flaccid paralysis of all skeletal muscles, absence of all spinal reflexes, absence of all cutaneous sensation, absence of all proprioceptive sensations, transient urinary and fecal retention); neck and back pain, which may radiate; decreased sensory level; obvious spinal deformity; limited body movement; and unconsciousness.

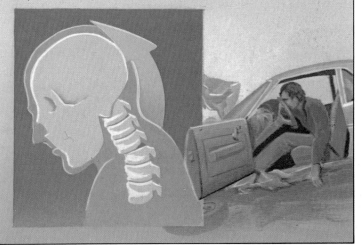

Spinal compression (Extreme compression of the spinal column)
Cause: Direct violence to the spine, such as in a fall from some distance in which the person lands on his feet or buttocks, causing compression of the lower thoracic or lumbar vertebrae. Compression may be severe enough to produce a fracture.
Signs and symptoms: Anterior cord injury syndrome (immediate, complete paralysis; hypesthesia and hypalgesia below the lesion); decreased vital signs; and signs of shock.

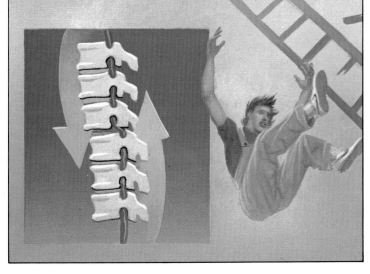

Diseases and disorders

Dealing with secondary neurologic injuries and complications

When we talk about a secondary neurologic injury or complication, we're referring to a disorder that develops as a result of a traumatic or nontraumatic primary injury. Secondary injuries and complications usually cause a rapid deterioration in your patient's condition. So, you'll need to quickly recognize changes in your patient's condition before they occur.

You'll also need to know how to care for your patient properly. Regardless of the cause of the secondary injury, follow these guidelines:
• Perform accurate and complete assessments when doing neurochecks. Document all your findings completely.
• Ensure a patent airway. Intubate the patient, if the doctor orders.
• Keep the patient's head elevated at all times to reduce venous pressure. In some cases, the doctor may place the patient on central venous pressure (CVP) monitoring.
• Monitor the patient for signs of increased intracranial pressure (ICP). If present, notify the doctor immediately. He may instruct you to prepare the patient for ICP monitoring or to administer osmotic diuretics, such as mannitol (Osmitrol*).
• Prepare the patient for diagnostic tests, such as a skull X-ray, computerized tomography (CT) scanning, and, in some cases, cerebral angiography.
• Prepare the patient and his family, if indicated, for surgery, such as twist drilling, the emergency burr hole procedure, or a craniotomy.
• Take seizure precautions.
• Observe any open wounds for signs of infection. Note any redness, temperature elevation, drainage, or odor. Notify the doctor immediately.

Then, study the chart below to learn more about the signs and symptoms of secondary injuries and complications.

Subdural hematoma

Epidural hematoma

Intracerebral hematoma

Subarachnoid hematoma

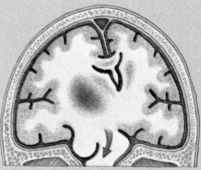
Uncal herniation

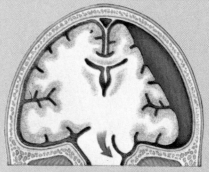
Tonsillar herniation

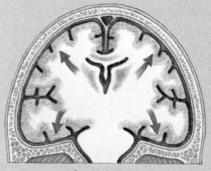
Cerebral edema

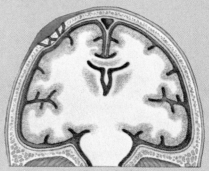
Localized infection

*Available in both the United States and in Canada

Problem	Cause	Implications	Signs and symptoms
Epidural hematoma Bleeding between the skull and dura mater in the epidural space	A tear in the wall of the middle meningeal artery, caused by a blunt blow to the head, as in a fall or a fight	Considered the most serious complication of head injury. Temporal lobe is forced down and inward, causing uncal herniation; may result in death.	Headache; ipsilateral pupil change; contralateral motor paralysis, such as hemiplegia on opposite side of hematoma; and unconsciousness, followed by period of alertness and lucidity, and then coma
Subdural hematoma Bleeding between the dura mater and the arachnoid into the subdural space	A laceration of the brain, with a tear in the arachnoid, allowing blood and cerebrospinal fluid to collect in subdural space; may also occur following a ruptured saccular aneurysm or intracerebral hemorrhage	May compress and further damage an already injured and edematous brain	Progressive change in level of consciousness; lateralizing changes (hemiparesis, ipsilateral pupil change, extraocular eye movement paralysis); irritability, confusion; positive Babinski response; and seizures
Subarachnoid hematoma Bleeding in the subarachnoid space	Injury to a surface vessel in the subarachnoid space	Bleeding may occur immediately or be delayed. Effects are similar to symptoms for ruptured aneurysm. May cause a *secondary* rise in ICP.	Sudden, violent headache; dizziness; vertigo; nausea, vomiting; drowsiness; sweating; and chills
Intracerebral hematoma Bleeding directly into the brain tissue	A cerebrum surface laceration following a penetrating or contrecoup skull injury. May be seen in hemorrhagic disorders.	May occur at impact site or some distance from initial injury. Contributes to the development of a subdural hematoma.	Increased intracranial pressure signs; headache; hemiplegia on opposite side from bleeding; dizziness; vomiting; and seizures
Uncal herniation (transtentorial herniation) Lateral displacement of the brain's medial structures	Medial portion of temporal lobe slipping across the tentorium into the posterior fossa, caused by an expanding lesion of temporal lobe or a lateral extracerebral lesion	Exerts pressure on the third cranial nerve and eventually the brain stem	Third nerve palsy (ipsilateral loss of direct reaction to light; ipsilateral ptosis; ipsilateral loss of medial rectus muscle movement; contralateral loss of consensual reaction to light; pupil is small at first, then becomes progressively larger and fixed); upper motor neuron involvement (motor paralysis affecting functionally-related group muscles; jackknife spasticity; hyperactive deep tendon reflexes in involved limbs; loss of cutaneous abdominal and cremasteric reflexes on paralyzed side; presence of Babinski response on paralyzed side; atrophy and fasciculations of involved muscles); loss of doll's eye reflex; decerebrate rigidity; hyperthermia; and other vital function disturbances, such as ataxic respiration pattern
Tonsillar herniation (medullary cone or cerebellar tonsillar herniation) Downward displacement of the brain's medial structures	Cerebellar tonsils pressing on the medulla, caused by an expanding lesion of the hemispheres or a centrally-located extracerebral lesion	May lead to medullary collapse and death	Altered level of consciousness; nuchal rigidity; upper motor neuron involvement (see above); respiratory changes (frequent sighs and yawns, leading to Cheyne-Stokes pattern and central neurogenic hyperventilation); decorticate posturing, progressing to decerebrate posturing; positive Babinski response; bilateral pupil enlargement; wide fluctuation in body temperature; and medullary collapse (flaccidity, respiration and/or circulatory collapse)
Cerebral edema Increased water content of white brain matter	Cerebral trauma; expanding lesions	May lead to increased tissue volume	Headache; dizziness, blurred vision; nausea; seizure; and signs of uncal or tonsillar herniation (late sign)
Localized infection Invasion and multiplication of microorganisms at injury site	Entrance of microorganisms into brain tissue through open head injury	Local cellular injury may spread to central nervous system, causing septicemia and bacteremia, which may result in death	Chills, fever; headache; convulsions; nuchal rigidity; stupor, and coma

Diseases and disorders

Traumatic head injuries: nursing considerations

What steps should you take to care for a patient with a traumatic head injury? Whether you're at the scene of an accident or in a hospital emergency department, basic care, as outlined here, stays the same.
- Ensure a patent airway.
- Assess your patient's total condition. He may have accompanying injuries to other organs which may go unnoticed.
- Position the patient correctly. Always assume the patient with a traumatic head injury also has a cervical spinal injury. Consequently, handle his head and neck with care, and immobilize them using proper equipment.
- Never remove a penetrating object from the head or back. Instead, immobilize it with gauze and tape.
- Perform a neurocheck. Observe the patient's level of consciousness for signs of deterioration. Monitor vital signs, watching especially for the signs and symptoms of shock. Maintain the patient's normal body temperature. Watch for the signs and symptoms of infection.
- Reorient your patient to person, time, and place.
- Control restlessness and pain with analgesics, such as promazine hydrochloride (Sparine*). *Never* give narcotics to an unconscious patient unless ordered.
- Prevent further complications by making sure the treatment of one disorder doesn't make another disorder worse.
- Check for nuchal rigidity. If present, notify the doctor.
- Observe the patient for cerebrospinal fluid leakage or bleeding from all cranial orifices.
- Observe the patient for signs of increased intracranial pressure.
- Take seizure precautions.
- Prevent the patient from straining when having a bowel movement. Give him stool softeners, if necessary.
- Document everything you've done in your nurses' notes.

Traumatic spinal injuries: nursing considerations

Your patient has suffered a traumatic injury to his vertebral column. Take every precaution to ensure that his injury doesn't become worse and involve the spinal cord. To provide him with proper health care, perform these basic steps:
- Ensure a patent airway. Intubate and suction, as necessary.
- Keep an emergency tracheotomy tray near the patient's bedside.
- Keep the patient in a supine position. Don't allow him to sit up.
- To prevent movement of the patient's spine when transporting, place him on a fracture board. Support the patient's head and neck at all times. Maintain firm, manual, longitudinal head traction during movement. Logroll him to ensure spinal alignment.
- Prevent head rotation by placing sandbags on both sides of the patient's head.
- Assess your patient for additional injuries.
- Watch for signs of shock. If hypotension develops, correct this condition by elevating the patient's legs and starting an I.V., as ordered. Carefully monitor the I.V. flow rate. (If patient's in spinal shock, fluid overload could be dangerous.)
- Perform neurochecks, as directed or as needed.
- Observe for signs of spinal shock syndrome (the total—but temporary—loss of sensory, motor, autonomic, and reflex activity *below* the level of the spinal cord injury). These signs include: complete flaccid paralysis of all muscles; absence of all spinal reflexes; absence of all cutaneous sensation; absence of all proprioceptive sensation; and transient urinary and fecal retention. If you observe any of these signs, notify the doctor immediately.
- Provide emotional support to the patient and his family.

*Available in both the United States and in Canada

Nurses' guide to nontraumatic neurologic disorders

How do you care for a patient with a nontraumatic neurologic disorder? That depends on the type of disorder, its rate of progression, and the patient's physical and mental condition. As you know, most nontraumatic disorders cause long-term, irreversible damage. Some disorders require surgery, while others necessitate radical changes in the patient's lifestyle.

You'll also need to help your patient and his family understand and cope with his disorder.

In addition to efficient nursing care, the doctor may order special care for your patient.

The chart that follows will familiarize you with some common nontraumatic neurologic disorders. In some cases, these disorders result in traumatic complications, so you'll also want to review the chart on pages 92 and 93. Understanding the causes of these disorders, and knowing how to recognize their signs and symptoms will better prepare you to care for your patient. For information on supportive nursing care, see pages 101 to 117.

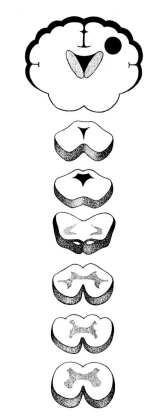

Intracranial tumor

Primary: (glioma glioblastoma, medulloblastoma, astrocytoma)
Possible cause
- Uncontrolled glial cell growth within the connective tissue of the brain

Characteristics
- Usually found in cerebral hemispheres; may also occur in adjacent brain locations, such as the cerebellum
- Not encapsulated

Secondary: (metastatic carcinoma or sarcoma)
Possible cause
- Uncontrolled cell growth

Characteristics
- Metastases from bronchogenic carcinoma, gastrointestinal or urinary tract tumors

Signs and symptoms
- Increased intracranial pressure symptoms; for example, headache, nausea, vomiting, vision impairment, papilledema
- Altered mental states (flattening of affect)
- Diminished intellectual ability, including confusion and decreased abstract thinking ability
- Dulling of recent and remote memory
- Shortened attention span
- Episodes of bizarre behavior
- Psychomotor seizures; for example, feelings of unreality, anger, detachment, fear, vertigo, déjà vu
- Bradycardia, progressing to cardiac arrest
- Respiratory changes, progressing to apnea
- Hypertension, progressing to hypotension
- Hyperthermia in the absence of infection

Extracranial tumor

Meningeal (meningioma)
Possible cause
- Uncontrolled tissue growth in the meninges

Characteristics
- Result of arachnoid granulation
- May occur in saggital sinus, central fissure, lateral fissure, sella turcica, and cerebellopontile angle
- Easily seen on X-ray because of calcification

Signs and symptoms
- Increased intracranial pressure
- Saggital region tumor: localized brain swelling
- Medial sphenoid ridge tumor: retrobulbar optic neuritis, central scotoma, optic atrophy on side of lesion, papilledema on opposite side of lesion
- Olfactory groove tumor: bilateral or unilateral anosmia

Cranial nerve (neuroma)
Possible cause
- Uncontrolled tissue growth originating at a cranial nerve root

Characteristics
- Usually occurs at eighth cranial nerve root (acoustic neuroma)
- May involve fifth cranial nerve

Signs and symptoms
- Ipsilateral hearing loss (partial or total)
- Hearing loss may be associated with tinnitus
- Vertigo
- Paresthesia and facial numbness with involvement of fifth cranial nerve

Posterior fossa (ependymoma, medulloblastoma)
Possible cause
- Ependymoma: glioma developing from ependymal cell lining of ventricles
- Medulloblastoma: glioma peculiar to the infratentorial compartment

Characteristics
- Ependymoma usually occurs along fourth ventricular pathway
- Medulloblastoma always found in the cerebellum

Signs and symptoms
- Headache (localized behind the ear or suboccipital region, more prominent on the side of the tumor), insidious on onset, usually worse in the morning, may be relieved by vomiting
- Patient may carry his head rotated toward the side where tumor's located
- Cranial nerve palsy
- Cerebellar signs; for example, ipsilateral ataxia, intention tremor, staggering gait, dysmetria, hypotonia
- Nystagmus

Neurovascular

Cerebrovascular accident (CVA)
Possible cause
- Narrowing or complete occlusion of one of the blood vessels supplying the brain

Characteristics
- May result from hypertension or arteriosclerosis

Signs and symptoms
- Speech disturbances
- Seizure
- Coma
- Nuchal rigidity
- Fever
- Hypertension
- Abnormal cardiac rhythms
- Peripheral and retinal vessel sclerosis
- Memory impairment
- Paralysis
- Increased intracranial pressure
- Visual impairment
- Dizziness

Cerebral ischemia
Possible cause
- Generalized or localized prolonged reduction in blood flow

Characteristics
- May result from atherosclerosis of intracranial and extracranial arteries; cerebral arterial vasoconstriction associated with migraine headaches; cerebral emboli; rheumatic heart disease, myocardial infarction (MI), or atrial fibrillation; subacute bacterial endocarditis; dissecting aortic arch aneurysm; cerebral hypoxia from cardiopulmonary insufficiency, pulmonary emboli or carbon monoxide poisoning

Signs and symptoms
- Visual, auditory, or vestibular disturbances
- Various motor and sensory disturbances
- Headache
- Slowing of mental processes
- Seizures

Cerebral infarction
Possible cause
- Cerebral necrosis from ischemia

Characteristics
- May result from neural cell swelling and disintegration
- Alterations in arterial system from heart to brain (atherosclerosis)
- Disruptions of brain's venous drainage system
- Decrease in blood viscosity and decrease in oxygen-carrying capacity of blood

Signs and symptoms
- Same as for cerebral ischemia

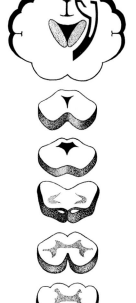
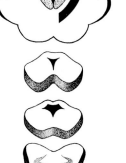

Diseases and disorders

Nurses' guide to nontraumatic neurologic disorders continued

Intracranial hemorrhage

Arteriovenous anomaly (arteriovenous fistulas, malformations, cavernous angiomas)
Possible cause
- Malformation allowing arterial blood to mingle with venous blood, without common capillaries

Characteristics
- Congenital

Signs and symptoms
- See arterial aneurysm

Arterial aneurysm (saccular, fusiform, mycotic, dissecting)
Possible cause
- A blood-filled sac (formed by arterial wall dilation) that's affected by degenerative changes and constant stress of blood flow

Characteristics
- May be congenital
- Saccular: found at arterial bifurcations at or near the circle of Willis; produces signs and symptoms when rupture occurs
- Fusiform: usually found on basilar or carotid artery; rarely hemorrhages; may press cranial nerve
- Mycotic: found at multiple locations; usually affects smaller branches of middle cerebral artery; may rupture eventually. Produced by septic emboli, usually associated with bacterial endocarditis.
- Dissecting: may be associated with saccular aneurysms; usually rare

Signs and symptoms
- Sudden, violent, severe headache
- Dizziness
- Nausea, vomiting
- Sweating, chills
- Alteration in consciousness level
- Irritability, photophobia, nuchal rigidity
- Severe neck and back pain
- Paralysis or paresis
- Speech disorders
- Visual disturbances; for example, diplopia, and vision loss
- Blood in cerebrospinal fluid following a lumbar or cisternal puncture distinguishes intracranial hemorrhage from cerebral infarct

Intracerebral tumor hemorrhage
Possible cause
- Bleeding from intracerebral primary or secondary tumors

Characteristics
- Most common in rapidly-growing, highly-vascular tumors; for example, metastatic bronchogenic carcinoma with brain metastasis

Signs and symptoms
- See arterial aneurysm

Hypertensive vascular disease
Possible cause
- Thickening and degeneration of cerebral arteriolae

Characteristics
- Results from hypertension
- Degeneration may lead to arteriole necroses and rupture
- Rupture and hemorrhage occurrence more common in cerebrum, but may occur anywhere in brain

Signs and symptoms
- See arterial aneurysm

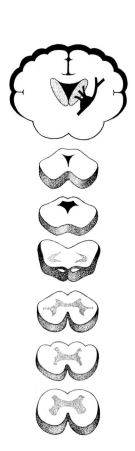

Infectious

Meningitis
Possible cause
- Multiplication of gram-negative *Neisseria meningitidis* in blood stream

Characteristics
- May lead to fulminant septicemia with meningeal involvement, capillary endothelial damage, vessel wall inflammation, necrosis, and thrombosis

Signs and symptoms
- Rash of varying severity
- Sepsis; for example, chills; low blood pressure; rapid, shallow respirations; overwhelming bacteremia
- Neck and back pain
- Stiff neck, retraction of head
- Hyperirritability
- Increased intracranial pressure
- Cheyne-Stokes respiratory pattern, leading to possible coma

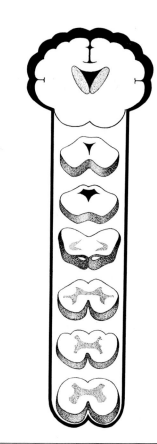

Encephalitis
Possible cause
- Brain inflammation

Characteristics
- Usually from arthropod-borne virus, exanthematous disease, vaccine, drug toxicity, or poisoning

Signs and symptoms
- Fever
- General malaise
- Sore throat
- Nausea, vomiting
- Lethargy
- Stiff neck
- Seizures
- Tremors
- Exaggerated deep tendon reflexes
- Spastic paralysis
- Cranial nerve paralysis
- Stupor or coma

Brain abscess
Possible cause
- Pus formation in brain substances

Characteristics
- May result from infection, or from extension of adjacent primary infection
- May be found in primary injuries of the middle ear; face; scalp; skull; mastoid and paranasal sinuses

Signs and symptoms
- Acute or subacute febrile illness accompanied by headache
- Localized neurologic disturbance
- Increased intracranial pressure

Guillain-Barré syndrome
Possible cause
- Inflammation and subsequent demyelination of nerve endings

Characteristics
- May result from hypersensitivity or autoimmune response to an inflammatory reaction
- May develop 1 to 2 weeks after a mild upper respiratory infection or gastroenteritis, or after administration of vaccines; for example, influenza vaccine

Signs and symptoms
- Lower extremity weakness progressing to upper extremities and face
- Total flaccid paralysis including respiratory muscles
- Facial diplegia
- Dysphagia
- Paresthesia of toes and fingers

Demyelinating

Multiple sclerosis (MS)
Possible cause
- Multifocal areas of demyelination, diffusely scattered throughout central nervous system (CNS)

Characteristics
- Periods of remission or exacerbation

Signs and symptoms
- Weakness and possible paralysis in one or more limbs
- Tremor
- Ataxia
- Abnormal ocular motor function (strabismus)
- Decreased perception to pain, touch, or temperature
- Charcot's triad (nystagmus, intention tremor, staccato speech)
- Diplopia
- Dizziness
- Cerebellar ataxia
- Mental changes (apathy, euphoria, inattentiveness)

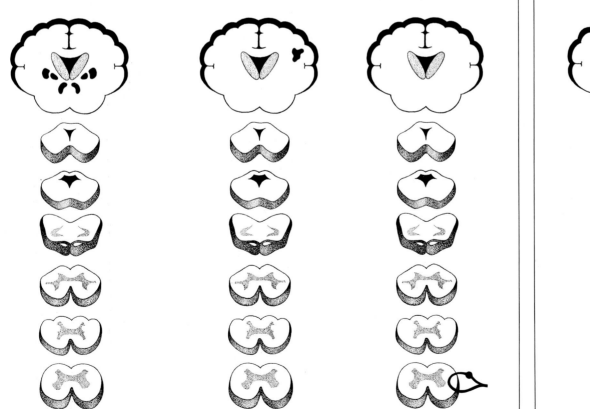
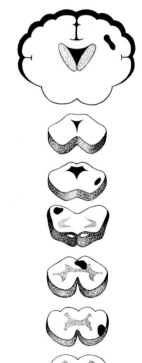

Diseases and disorders

Nurses' guide to nontraumatic neurologic disorders continued

Miscellaneous

Myasthenia gravis
Possible cause
- Neuromuscular disease

Characteristics
- Fluctuating weakness of certain voluntary muscles, especially those innervated by cranial nerves originating in the brain stem (ocular, facial, lingual, and masticatory)
- May be caused by autoimmune deficiency

Signs and symptoms
- Abnormal fatigue
- Progressive muscle weakness
- Extraocular weakness producing ptosis
- Diplopia
- Progressive, compromised ability to speak and swallow after prolonged activity
- High-pitched nasal voice
- Blank, expressionless face

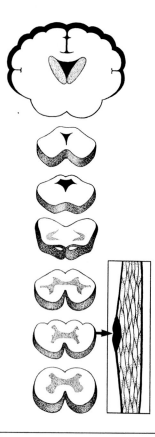

Epilepsy (seizure disorder, or idiopathic epilepsy)
Possible cause
- Abnormal and excessive discharge of neurons in various brain areas

Characteristics
- Recurrent seizures (when no extracerebral neurologic cause for their appearance exists) may occur as a symptom of cerebral ischemia, metabolic disturbances such as electrolyte imbalance (low K+ or low glucose level), drug withdrawal, or a brain lesion (tumor, trauma, or infection) producing an irritable focus

Signs and symptoms
- Grand mal: aura followed by a loss of consciousness; skeletal muscles undergo rigid extended (tonic) contractures; may be associated with cyanosis and/or dyspnea; alternate contraction and relaxation (clonic) movements; loss of bowel and bladder control.
- Petit mal: myoclonic or akinetic episodes with brief memory lapses, sudden vacant expression, cessation of motor activity, and loss of muscle tone.
- Jacksonian: limited seizure without consciousness loss.
- Psychomotor: focal motor seizure without consciousness loss; incoherent speech; turning of head and eyes; lip smacking; clouding of consciousness, and amnesia.
- Status epilepticus; rapid repetitive recurrence of any type of seizure without recovery between attacks. Patient remains unconscious and has continuous seizures with tonic and clonic fluctuations, incontinence, severely disturbed breathing, high fever, excessive diaphoresis, and elevated blood pressure. *Note:* Status epilepticus requires immediate emergency treatment.

Parkinson's disease (parkinsonism, paralysis agitans, or shaking palsy)
Possible cause
- Degeneration within the nuclear masses of extrapyramidal system

Characteristics
- May be associated with post encephalitis, atherosclerosis, neurosyphilis, carbon monoxide poisoning, or head trauma
- May result from excessive use of phenothiazides, such as chlorpromazine hydrochloride (Thorazine); reserpine (Elserpine) or haloperidol (Haldol*)

Signs and symptoms
- Tremors, usually accompanied with pill-rolling movements of thumb against fingers
- Dyskinesia (impaired voluntary activity resulting in fragmentary or incomplete movements; for example, stiffness, or shuffling short-stepped gait)
- Mood and personality disturbances
- Low-pitched, slow, monotonous speech
- Drooling

Cranial and peripheral nerves

Trigeminal neuralgia (tic douloureux)
Possible cause
- Direct nerve pressure

Characteristics
- Affects sensory function of fifth cranial nerve

Signs and symptoms
- Sharp stabbing facial pain in one or more of the nerve's three branches (ophthalmic, maxillary, and mandibular)
- Pain may be triggered by cold, wind, touch, shaving, swallowing, chewing, or talking

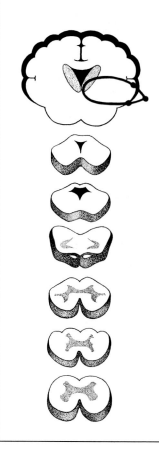

Acute labyrinthitis
Possible causes
• Organisms, such as those causing acute febrile diseases, erode bony labyrinth, allowing bacteria to enter from middle ear
• Toxic drug ingestion, alcohol abuse, allergy, severe fatigue
Characteristics
• Affects ear's semicircular canal system
• Disease of eighth cranial nerve
Signs and symptoms
• Severe sudden vertigo
• Nausea
• Sudden equilibrium disturbance
• Sudden nystagmus
• Photophobia

Carpal tunnel syndrome
Possible cause
• Inflammation or fibrosis of tendon sheaths passing through carpal tunnel results in edema and median nerve compression of wrist
Characteristics
• Occurs spontaneously, or follows injury or disease
Signs and symptoms
• Localized pain; for example, weakness, burning, numbness, or tingling in one or both hands
• Paresthesia affecting thumb, forefinger, and middle finger

Bell's Palsy
Possible cause
• Inflammation, affecting muscles of expression on one side of face
• No pathological cause for facial paralysis
Characteristics
• Peripheral paralysis of seventh cranial nerve (affects motor function)
Signs and symptoms
• On affected side, upward movement of the eyeball when closing eye, slight lag of eyelid on closing, drooping of the mouth, flattening of nasolabial fold

Headaches

Vascular (classic migraine; common migraine; cluster migraine)
Possible cause
• Early neurologic symptoms may be from vasoconstriction; later symptoms (intense throbbing headache) may be from dilation of extracranial and intracranial branches of the external carotid artery

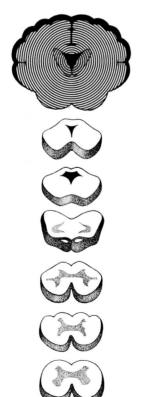

Characteristics
• Classic migraine: onset occurs in unilateral, temporal, or frontal areas; high hereditary incidence; personality factors may contribute; usually periodic and recurrent
• Common migraine: may be unilateral and spreading; high hereditary incidence; may be relieved by pregnancy or illness; gradual onset, episodic; increases with each life crisis
• Cluster migraine (histamine headaches): excruciatingly painful, unilateral headaches that occur for a few days, weeks, or even months (clusters) followed by remission with no symptoms for months
Signs and symptoms:
• Classic migraine: transient visual field defects; transient paralysis; paralysis of an arm or leg; confusion (may subside as pain begins); photophobia; nausea; vomiting; irritability; constipation; chills; sweating
• Common migraine: vague psychic disturbances for several hours or days before headache begins; nausea; vomiting; chills; nasal stuffiness; localized or generalized edema; diuresis
• Cluster migraine: intense throbbing pain arising high in the nostril and spreading to one side of the forehead, around and behind the eye on the affected side; nasal and ocular lacrimation may also occur on affected side; skin may redden on affected side; nasal congestion

Muscular (tension headache)
Possible causes
• Long sustained skeletal muscle contracture around the face, scalp, neck, and upper back
• Vasodilation of associated cranial arteries may also contribute to the irritability of the involved muscles and head pain
Characteristics
• May be unilateral or bilateral; pain frequently occurs in occipital and upper cervical areas and radiates over the top of the head
• Headaches may be unrelieved for weeks, months, and years
• Headaches are fleeting, but recurrent
• Onset is gradual
• May be associated with depression and anxiety
Signs and symptoms
• Feelings of tightness, pressure, drawing sensation, or fullness; pain may be localized or may vary in intensity and location
• Dizziness, tinnitus, lacrimation
• Contracted muscles may be palpated with localized painful areas
• Exposure to cold may precipitate or aggravate the headache
• Nausea and vomiting (usually late signs and symptoms)

Diseases and disorders

Intracranial tumors: recognizing signs and symptoms

Intracranial tumors are one of the most common disorders affecting the nervous system. When left untreated, these tumors—whether benign or malignant—may be potentially fatal. So, recognizing signs and symptoms is crucial to early tumor identification and treatment.

On pages 96 to 99, we reviewed generalized signs and symptoms associated with any expanding brain mass. But a patient with an intracranial tumor also faces localized signs and symptoms; for example, focal weakness, and sensory, language, coordination, and visual disorders. These signs and symptoms vary depending on tumor location, but result from *irritation*, *compression*, and *destruction* of *specific* brain tissue. They may occur at any time and cannot be predicted.

Learn how to identify intracranial tumor location by familiarizing yourself with the localized signs and symptoms detailed in the following illustration.

Frontal lobe
Changes in personality or behavior; intellectual dysfunction; hemiparesis; aphasia (dominant hemisphere); and focal motor seizures

Cerebrum
Generalized seizures; and neurologic dysfunction

Parietal lobe
Hemisensory impairment; visual disturbances, such as inferior quadrantic hemianopia; and focal sensory seizures

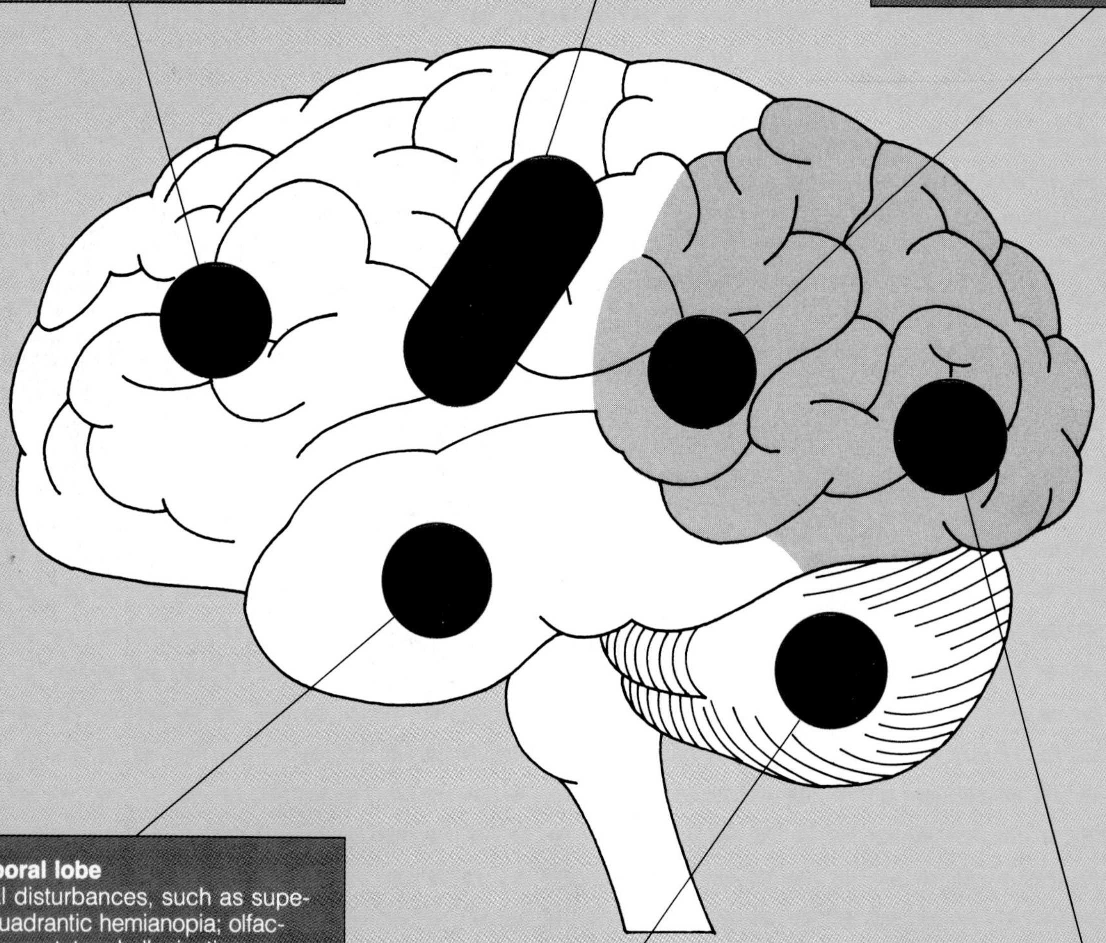

Temporal lobe
Visual disturbances, such as superior quadrantic hemianopia; olfactory or gustatory hallucinations; psychomotor seizures; for example, detachment, anger, sense of unreality, déjà vu, vertigo; memory defects; and nominal aphasia (dominant hemisphere)

Cerebellum
Ataxia; nystagmus; dysmetria; and unsteady gait

Occipital lobe
Visual disturbances, such as homonymous hemianopia; aura flashes of light; and seizures

Nursing care

So far in this section, we've discussed how to recognize and manage the signs and symptoms of traumatic and nontraumatic disorders. In the following pages, we'll take a look at how to provide day-to-day nursing care for your patient with a neurologic disorder.

To begin, we'll provide some care guidelines for a patient scheduled for neurosurgery. Then, we'll tell you how to provide patient care during a seizure and how to document your patient's seizure properly. In addition, we'll familiarize you with post-traumatic epilepsy, and you'll learn how to insert an artificial airway.

No matter what type of neurologic disorder your patient has, most of your nursing care will be directed toward providing patient comfort and preventing complications. That's why we'll review how to suction your patient, how to use a hyper-hypothermia blanket, and how to perform suprapubic catheterization.

Of course, you'll also want to know about these special challenges:
• dealing with daily care complications
• providing emotional support to the patient and his family
• managing concussions.

You can find out about these procedures and more by reading the following pages.

Caring for a patient scheduled for neurosurgery

Is your patient scheduled for neurosurgery? If so, you'll be responsible for preparing him and his family for surgery, and for his care afterwards.

Begin by following these guidelines:
Preoperative care
• Make sure the patient's received preoperative patient teaching. Answer any questions he or his family may have.
• Administer preoperative bowel care cautiously, and only as ordered. Instruct your patient to avoid straining during bowel movements. As you know, straining elevates intracracranial pressure.
• Withhold food and fluids, as ordered.
• Perform routine neurochecks.
• Ask the doctor if he wants to change to a parenteral route to administer special medications, such as anticonvulsants and sedatives. Be sure the dosage has been adjusted.
• Make sure your patient's signed a consent form.
• Before administering any narcotics or hypnotics, double-check the order with the doctor. These medications may be contraindicated in patients scheduled for neurosurgery.
Immediately before surgery
• Prep the patient, as ordered. This may include applying scalp medications, or shaving the operative site.
• Have the patient urinate. Or, insert an indwelling (Foley) catheter, if the doctor orders.
• Perform a complete neurocheck, and document the results in your notes. That way, you'll have a preoperative baseline with which to compare your postop neurochecks.
• Apply antiembolism stockings, as ordered.

After surgery, make your patient as comfortable as possible. Place the patient in semi-Fowler's position. *Caution:* Never lower the patient's head below heart level. Doing so increases intracranial pressure.

Monitor your patient's progress by performing neurochecks frequently. *Remember:* Only take your patient's temperature rectally. Oral temperature readings are contraindicated following neurosurgery. As you observe and assess your patient, follow these guidelines:
• Be alert for signs of possible complications, such as cerebral swelling, cerebrospinal fluid (CSF) drainage, or bleeding. If you see any of these signs, notify the doctor.
• Check the patient's dressing frequently. Reinforce the dressing, as needed. Notify the doctor if the dressing seems tight, or you see abnormal swelling, bleeding, or CSF drainage.
• Turn and position your patient for secretion drainage. To prevent bleeding or increased intracranial pressure, never suction your patient or encourage him to cough, unless you have a written order from the doctor.
• Administer oxygen or mechanical ventilation, as ordered.
• Give medications such as anticonvulsants and diuretics, as ordered.
• Double-check any order for a narcotic. Heavily sedating a patient following neurosurgery may cause complications, such as respiratory distress, and may be contraindicated.
• Closely monitor intake and output.
• Administer fluids I.V. until ordered otherwise. *Do not give fluids orally without an order.* Make sure you explain this to the patient's family.
• Routinely check to be sure the I.V. is set at the prescribed rate. Keep in mind that rapid administration of fluids I.V. increases intracranial pressure, or may produce left-sided heart failure.
• Never administer enemas, cathartics, or any bowel medications, unless ordered by the doctor.
• Explain to the patient why he should avoid straining during bowel movements or coughing episodes.

And finally, document everything in your notes.

Understanding post-traumatic epilepsy

As you should know, epilepsy's a disorder of the brain that causes recurrent paroxysmal attacks of unconsciousness, convulsive movements, and other motor or behavioral abnormalities.

Post-traumatic epilepsy can occur immediately after major or minor head injuries, though it more commonly happens months after the patient's dura mater has been penetrated and his underlying cortex lacerated, creating cerebromeningeal scar formation. That's why the patient must understand the importance of taking anticonvulsant medication for up to 2 years after the injury, as ordered by the doctor.

Occasionally, a patient may have a seizure from a complication, such as a hematoma, abscess, or meningitis, rather than from the injury itself.

The following measures will help prevent immediate post-traumatic epilepsy after a severe brain injury.
• If the patient has a depressed skull fracture, elevate his head.
• If the patient has a compound skull fracture, the doctor will debride the area. Then, he'll suture the dura mater to prevent infection and minimize the amount of scar formation.

Nursing care

Taking seizure precautions

Whenever you care for a patient with a head injury, you can minimize seizure risk by taking the following precautions:
• Administer anticonvulsant medications on time. Do not omit or increase medication.
• Be sure to use a rectal thermometer, not an oral one, on the seizure-prone patient.
• Pad side rails and headboard to protect him from injury.
• Keep the padded, long side rails in place if he has frequent or generalized seizures, or if he has severe muscle contractions.
• When a patient has an oral endotracheal tube in place, insert an airway to prevent the patient from occluding or biting the endotracheal tube during seizure activity, and to allow for suctioning.
• Keep suction equipment handy in case the patient's airway becomes clogged with oral secretions.
• Monitor the patient's cardiovascular and respiratory status closely to detect hypoxia which may lead to increased seizure activity.
• Provide emotional support to the patient and family.
• Accompany the seizure-prone patient when he takes a walk.

Nursing care during a seizure

Dealing with a seizure effectively involves both calm observation and quick action. Doing both tasks well is a challenge, but simply knowing *what* to do beforehand helps. When your patient has a seizure, take these actions:
• Stay with the patient and call for assistance.
• Lay the patient flat on the bed or floor. (Don't try to lift a patient onto a bed while he's having a seizure.) Then, try to turn him on his side.
• Loosen tight clothing; for example, his collar and belt.
• Move objects out of the way to protect his head and limbs from injury.
• Guide his movements, if possible, but don't restrain him.
• Don't force open clenched teeth.

Inserting an artificial airway

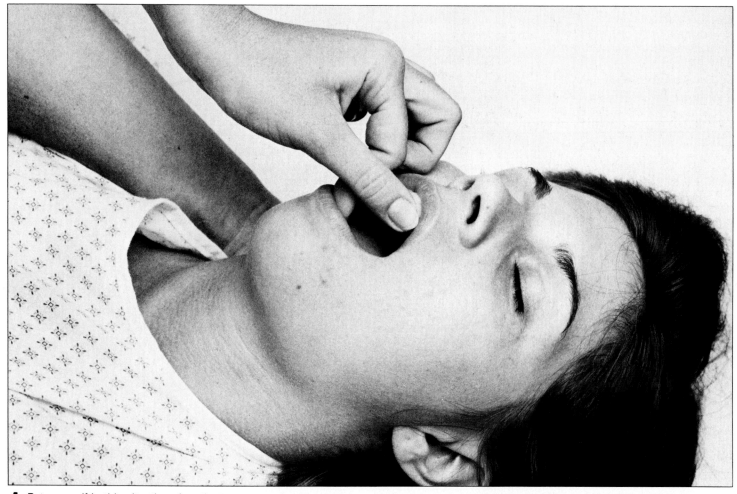

1 *Put yourself in this situation: A patient on your unit with a head injury suddenly appears confused and lethargic. You recognize this altered state of consciousness and realize that to prevent hypoxia, you must insert an artificial airway. Here's how: If the* patient's mouth is closed, immediately open it by using a crossed-finger technique, as shown here.
Remember: If you suspect cerebral or cervical spine injury, don't use a modified jaw thrust.

- Provide privacy, if possible.

After your patient's seizure, take these actions:

- Place him in bed, if he isn't already.
- Ensure a patent airway by turning him on his side to permit oral drainage. Check his level of consciousness. If it's depressed, insert an oral airway. Suction, as needed.
- If this is the patient's first seizure, notify the doctor immediately. If the patient has had seizures before, notify the doctor immediately only if the seizure activity is prolonged or the patient fails to regain consciousness.
- Check the patient for injury.
- Reorient and reassure the patient as necessary.
- Document everything in your nurses' notes.

Documenting a seizure

Immediately after your patient's seizure, record the answers to these questions:
- *Onset:* Was it sudden, or preceded by an aura? If preceded by an aura, have the patient describe what he experienced.
- *Duration:* What time did the seizure begin and end?
- *Frequency and number:* Did he have one seizure or several?
- *State of consciousness:* Was the patient unconscious? If so, for how long? Could you arouse him? Note any changes in consciousness.
- *Motor activity:* Where did the motor activity begin? What parts of his body were involved? Was there a pattern of progression to the activity? Describe his movements.
- *Eyes and tongue:* Did they deviate to one side? Did his pupils change in size, shape, equality, or in their reaction to light?
- *Teeth:* Were they clenched or open?
- *Respirations:* What was his respiratory rate and quality? Was he cyanotic?
- *Body activities:* Did he have incontinence, vomiting, salivation, or oral bleeding?
- *Drug response:* If any drugs were administered during the seizure, how did the patient respond? Did the seizure cease? Did it worsen?
- *Seizure awareness:* Is the patient aware of what happened? Did he immediately go into a deep sleep following the seizure? Was he upset? Did he seem ashamed?

2 Now, insert the artificial airway in one of these two ways. The quickest way is this: Point the tip of the artificial airway toward the roof of her mouth. Gently advance the airway by rotating it 180°; then, slide it into place.

Don't be surprised if your patient gags at first. If she does, hold the airway in place without advancing it for a few seconds, until she relaxes.

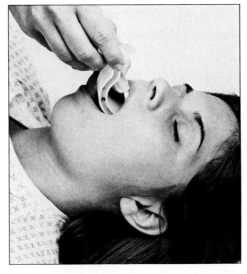

3 Here's another way to insert an artificial airway. Hold the tongue down with a tongue depressor, and guide the artificial airway over the back of the tongue until it's in position. (You'll find this method particularly easy to use with infants, because their tongues are flat.)

If your patient gags, hold the airway in place until she relaxes.

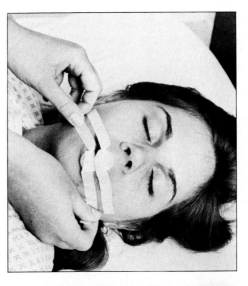

4 To keep the artificial airway from slipping out of place, tape two ½" adhesive strips across the top and bottom of the artificial airway, and secure it to the patient's cheeks.

Always make sure you've allowed enough room for suctioning.

5 Once the artificial airway is in place, logroll the patient, keeping her head and neck aligned, so she's positioned on her side. This will decrease the risk of aspiration if she vomits.

Document the date and time of airway insertion, as well as the patient's tolerance to the procedure.

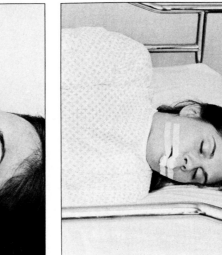

Nursing care

Suctioning your patient

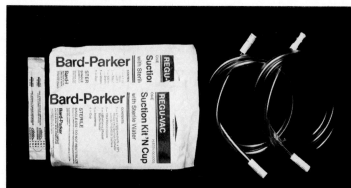

1 *Picture this: You're caring for 22-year-old Francis Zeller, who's unconscious. During the past 2 hours, she's had excessive oral secretions. Her doctor orders suctioning, as needed. Do you know how to perform this procedure properly? If you're unsure, follow these guidelines:*

Begin by gathering the equipment you'll need: two sterile suction kits (each containing a suction catheter, disposable basin, 4 oz. packet of sterile water, and a sterile glove); and two lengths of suction tubing. You'll also need a suction canister, a suction regulator, and a hand-held resuscitator. Remember, if the suction catheters you're using don't have control valves, obtain a sterile Y connector. Mount the suction canister on the wall.

Then, wash your hands thoroughly before proceeding.

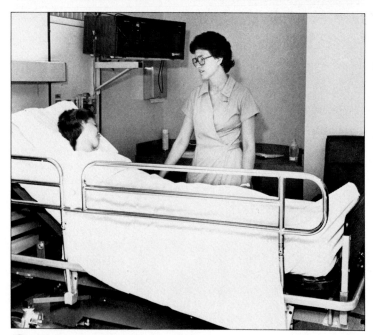

2 Explain the procedure to Ms. Zeller, and check to be sure the head of her bed is elevated, unless contraindicated.

■ *Nursing tip:* Ask the doctor to order a humidifier or vaporizer to be kept at the patient's bedside. The moisture produced by either of these units helps liquefy the patient's secretions, and makes suctioning less uncomfortable for her.

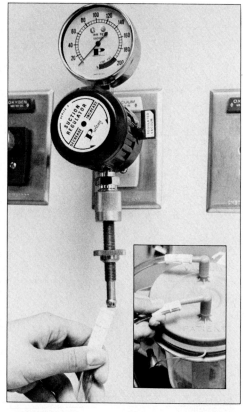

3 Attach one end of the suction tubing to the suction regulator.

[Inset] Attach the other end of the suction tubing to the suction canister.

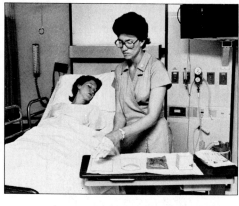

4 Using aseptic technique, open one suction kit. Put the sterile glove on the hand you'll be working with.

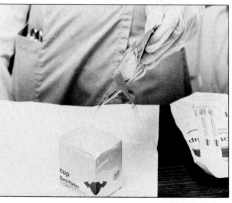

5 Open the packet of sterile water and pour it into the disposable basin, as shown. Be careful not to contaminate your gloved hand.

6 Next, use your gloved hand to pull the catheter from its wrapper.

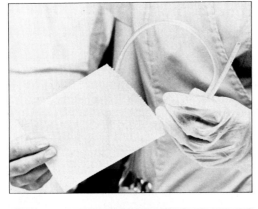

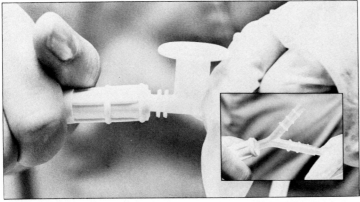

7 Holding the catheter in your gloved hand, attach the catheter's adapter to the suction tubing, as the nurse is doing here.
[Inset] If the catheter lacks a control valve, place a sterile Y connector on its distal end. Then, attach the Y connector to the suction tubing.

8 Prepare for suctioning by setting the suction regulator dial to low (20 mm Hg). Turn on the suction regulator. Next, dip the catheter in sterile water to lubricate it, making sure that you do not draw up water into the catheter.

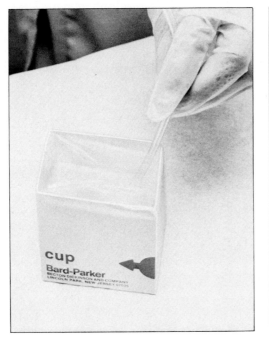

9 Now you're ready to begin suctioning Ms. Zeller's mouth. First, insert the catheter in her cheek areas without creating suction. Then, placing your thumb over the suction valve, drain secretions from her upper and lower jaws. Control suctioning by intermittently covering the valve with your thumb.

[Inset] If you're using a Y connector, intermittently cover the open end of the connector with your thumb.

Remember, you can also control suctioning by bending and pinching the catheter between your fingers.

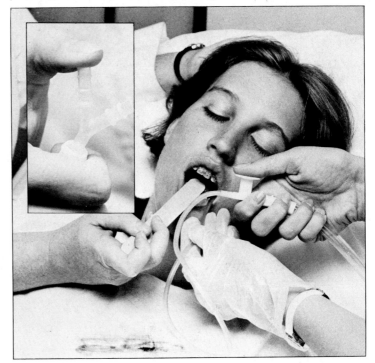

10 Suppose your patient has an artificial airway. Suction, as ordered by the doctor, through or alongside the airway, as shown in this illustration.

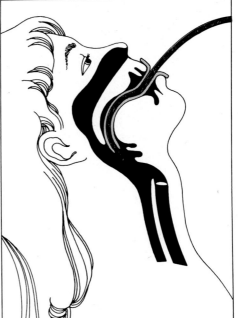

Nursing care

Suctioning your patient continued

11 Now you've finished suctioning Ms. Zeller's mouth. Use your ungloved hand to pull the glove inside out, and down over the catheter. Avoid touching your ungloved hand to either the outside of the glove or the catheter. Dispose of both in a wastebasket, as shown.

Important: Never use the same catheter to suction both the mouth and the trachea. Doing so may introduce oral bacteria into the patient's respiratory tract. Keep in mind that your patient's defense mechanisms are already compromised.

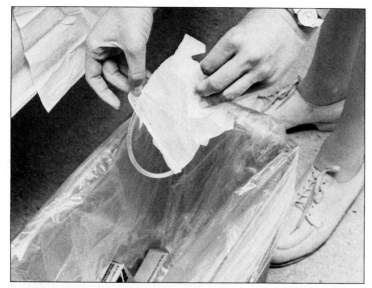

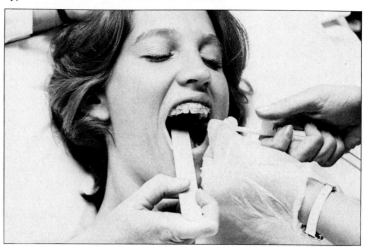

13 Gently insert the catheter into her pharynx. Be sure the catheter tip isn't pushed below the epiglottis.

Remember: Deep-suctioning a patient with a neurologic injury or disorder may cause gasping, or a rise in intracranial pressure.

Now, begin suctioning the patient. To do so, completely withdraw the catheter with a twirling movement as you apply intermittent suction. Remember, never move the catheter up and down rapidly, or you may traumatize your patient's tracheal mucosa. Rinse the catheter with sterile water each time you reinsert it.

Caution: To prevent hypoxia or possible cardiac arrest, minimize the length of time you'll be suctioning. If your patient is hypoxic, hyperventilate her before each reinsertion.

12 Now, you're ready to suction her pharynx, using the second sterile suction kit. Before you begin, hyperventilate your patient with 100% oxygen, using a hand-held resuscitator with a reservoir. Oxygenating your patient will prevent possible cardiac arrhythmias caused by hypoxia.

Then, repeat steps 4 through 8, maintaining aseptic technique.

14 To ensure removal of all secretions, turn your patient's head first to one side, then to the other as you suction. Then, position her head forward and suction.

When you've completed the procedure, again hyperventilate Ms. Zeller with oxygen. Dispose of the catheter and glove as described in step 11. Thoroughly wash your hands.

Document the suctioning procedure in your nurses' notes. Record the amount, consistency, and color of the secretions; presence of blood in the secretions; and how well your patient tolerated the procedure.

Performing mouth care

The patient with a neurologic injury or disorder may need you to perform the mouth care he's used to performing himself. To provide him with this care, do the following tasks at least three times a day.

Gather the following equipment and place it at the patient's bedside: a mouth-care kit containing toothbrush, two cups, and tongue depressors. You'll also need hydrogen peroxide solution, water, lip moisturizer, a flashlight, bite stick, bed-saver pad, emesis basin, gloves, and a 20 cc syringe with soft rubber extension. To perform mouth care, follow these guidelines:
• Position the patient on his side with the head of his bed elevated, unless contraindicated. Put a bed-saver pad under the patient's head and shoulders.
• Fill one cup with 50% water, 50% hydrogen peroxide solution, and a small amount of mouthwash. Fill the other cup with water. Put a small amount of toothpaste on the toothbrush and place it, along with the bite stick, on the bed-saver pad.
• Turn on the suction machine and keep it on, with the suction catheter handy at all times, in case your patient's airway becomes obstructed.

• Wash your hands thoroughly and put on clean gloves.
• Inspect the oral cavity using the flashlight and tongue depressor. Note the condition of his teeth, gums, tongue, palate, and lips. Observe for loose teeth, bleeding, discoloration, swelling, and ulcerations. Record your observations.
• Brush the patient's teeth and gums thoroughly, but gently. Next, brush his tongue and palate.
• Place the emesis basin at the side of his mouth and rest his cheek on the basin. Rinse his mouth thoroughly using the water, hydrogen peroxide solution, and mouthwash combination. At the same time, with your other hand, use the suction catheter to suction the mouth continuously.
• Thoroughly rinse the entire mouth with water and suction it dry. Wash and dry the patient's face. If your patient has an endotracheal tube in place, you'll also need to change the tape.
• Finally, apply water-soluble lip moisturizer, such as lemon and glycerine.
• Document your care, observations, and the patient's tolerance to the procedure, in your nurses' notes.

Using the Blanketrol® Hyper-Hypothermia blanket

1 *As you probably know, many patients with neurologic disorders experience extreme fluctuations in body temperature. These extreme fluctuations interfere with cerebral metabolism and can cause delirium, stupor, and coma. To help maintain your patient's temperature within the normal range, you may use a temperature-control system like the Blanketrol Hyper-Hypothermia system. In this photostory, you'll learn how to set up this equipment.*

Gather two Hyper-Hypothermia blankets, rectal probe, and Blanketrol machine, as shown. Make sure the blankets are prefilled with water. Then, check them for signs of leakage. If you see any damp spots, replace them before proceeding. In addition to the equipment shown here, you'll need nonallergenic tape, scissors, Skin-Prep™, and two disposable blanket covers, supplied by the manufacturer.

Lift the water reservoir cover and check the water level. The reservoir should be filled with distilled water ½" to 1" above

the copper tubing visible at the reservoir opening. If necessary, add more distilled water.

Note: To prevent bacterial growth, an antibacterial agent may be added to the water. Check the manufacturer's instructions for recommendations.

Now, make sure the master control toggle switch is in OFF position; then, plug the Servo controller panel into the Blanketrol machine. Insert the machine's three-prong plug into a properly-grounded outlet.

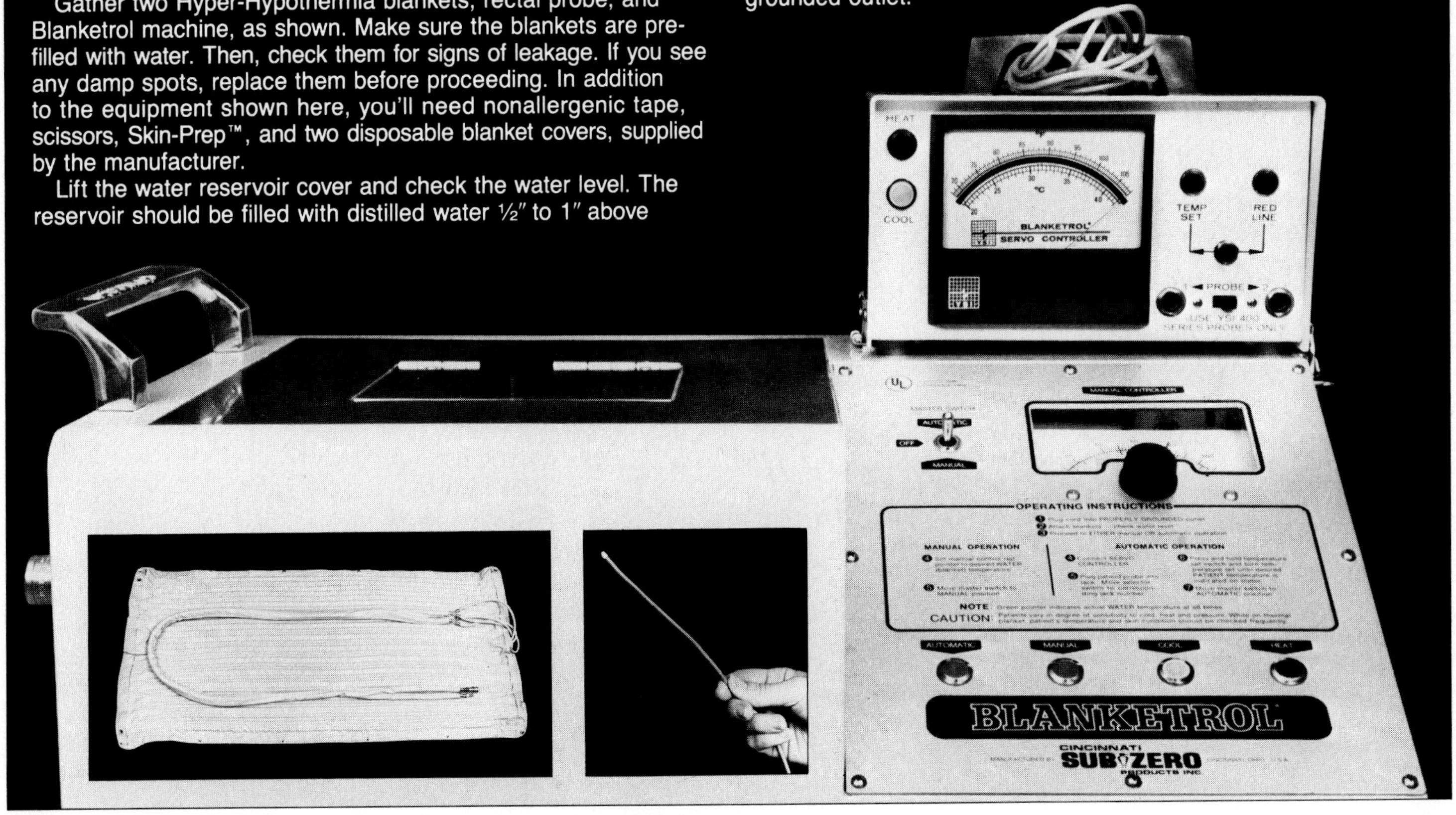

Nursing care

Using the Blanketrol® Hyper-Hypothermia blanket continued

2 Explain the equipment to the patient. Record his vital signs and perform a thorough neurocheck. This provides a baseline for assessing the patient's response to therapy.

Then, place one of the blankets alongside him, as the nurse has done here. Cover the blanket with a disposable blanket cover.

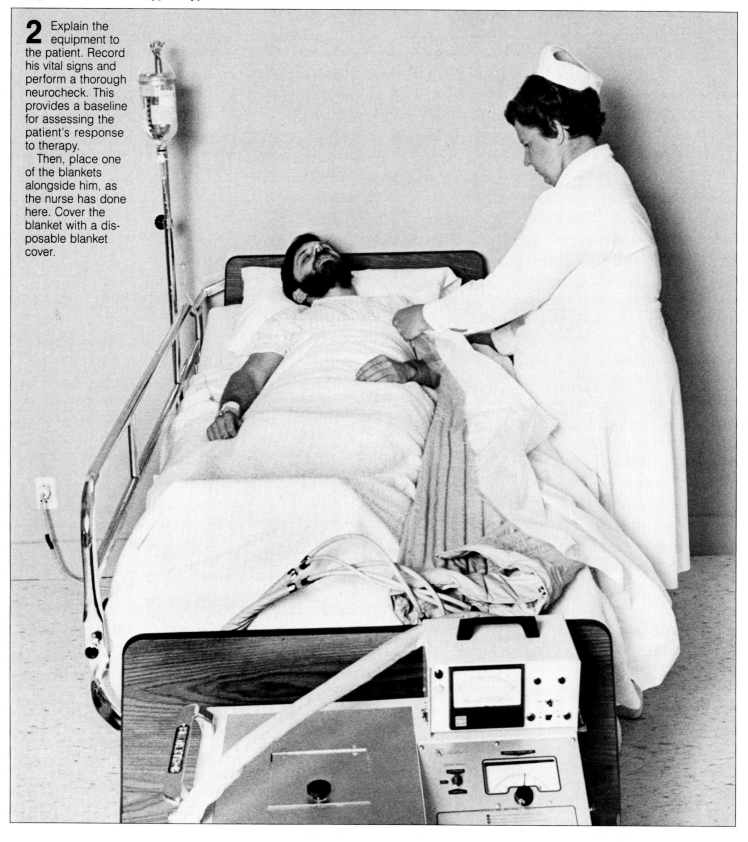

3 Turn the patient on his side, and position the blanket under him.

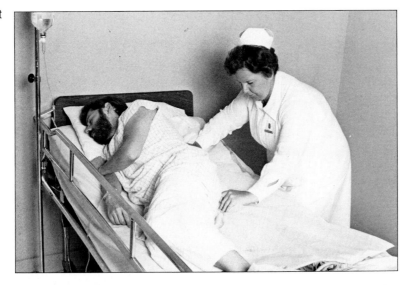

4 Now, insert the rectal probe. Advance it about 6″ into his rectum. Apply Skin-Prep to his leg or buttock before taping the probe there. *Note:* You may use a skin or esophageal probe instead of a rectal probe, depending on the patient's condition.

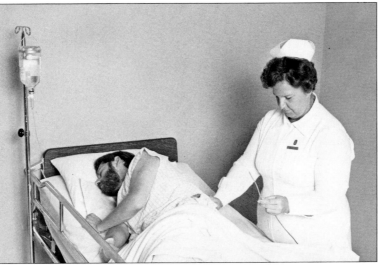

5 If you need to increase or decrease your patient's body temperature quickly, use the second Blanketrol blanket, as well. Place this one over him, as the nurse is doing here.
☎ *Nursing tip:* Disposable Blanketrol blankets are available to cover your patient. Because the disposable blankets are lightweight, your patient will be more comfortable.

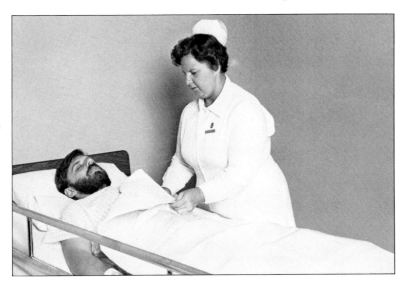

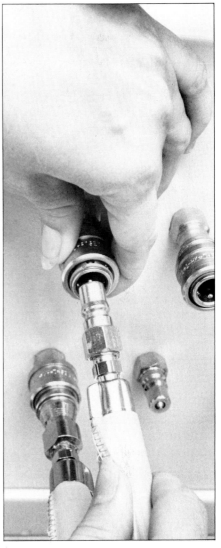

6 Now you're ready to connect the set of blanket cables for the blanket underneath the patient to the side of the Blanketrol machine. To do so, grasp the female adapter on the blanket cable and slide the collar backward. Push the female coupling over one of the male couplings on the lower left side of the Blanketrol machine. Let the collar return into place; then, pull the cable to assure a secure connection.

Next, slide the collar back on one of the machine's female couplings, as the nurse is doing here, and insert the cable's male adapter into it. Push in the cable's male adapter until you hear a click.

Repeat this procedure with the set of cables for the blanket that's on top of the patient (if you used one).

Nursing care

Using the Blanketrol® Hyper-Hypothermia blanket continued

7 Next, insert the probe's plug into one of the probe receptacles, as shown here. Choose the receptacle closest to your patient to alleviate pulling on the probe. Then, push the probe selector switch toward the probe receptacle that you're using.

To calibrate the Blanketrol unit, push the temperature/calibration toggle switch toward the right, and watch the patient temperature indicator needle. The needle should come to rest directly over the red line calibration checkpoint. If it doesn't, continue to hold the toggle switch and use your scissors to turn the screw labeled RED LINE, until the needle rests over the red line. Then, release the toggle switch.

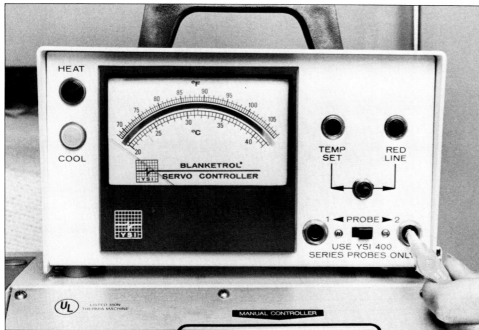

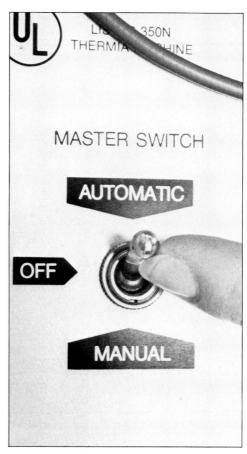

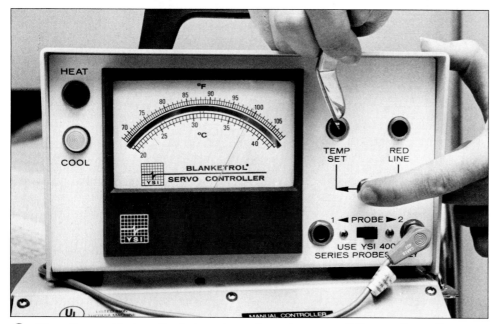

8 When the machine's calibrated, you're ready to set the temperature ordered for your patient. To do so, press the temperature/calibration toggle switch to the left, toward TEMP SET. If the needle reading isn't the same as the doctor ordered, adjust it by turning the TEMP SET screw until it is. Release the toggle switch.

9 Now, push the master control switch to the AUTOMATIC position. The automatic cycle indicator will light, and water will begin to circulate through the system. The automatic setting maintains the patient's temperature at the preset level. (Use the MANUAL setting to treat two patients at once. See the manufacturer's instructions for details.)

Check the patient's vital signs every half hour, until they're stable. Monitor his heart rate, and conduct neurochecks throughout treatment. At least once an hour, check the patient for signs of edema, inflammation, skin color changes, and other signs of burns or frostbite.

To discontinue blanket use, turn off the master control toggle switch, remove the rectal probe, and disconnect the machine's plug from the wall outlet. Then, remove the blankets from under and on top of the patient. Remove the disposable blanket covers. Disconnect the blanket cables from the side of the Blanketrol machine, and fold the cables inside the blankets. Store the hyper-hypothermia blankets following manufacturer's guidelines. If you're using disposable blankets, you may discard them.

Learning about autonomic dysreflexia

How much do you know about autonomic dysreflexia? Did you know that this life-threatening condition is triggered by *blocked afferent impulses* caused by a spinal lesion? Normally, on stimulation, sensory receptors in the bladder and bowel send impulses through the spinal cord to the brain. In patients with spinal cord injuries, however, these impulses are obstructed by the lesion. This blockage produces a reflex arteriolar spasm by way of the sympathetic ganglia of the nervous system. The resulting arteriole vasoconstriction immediately raises the patient's blood pressure.

Then, baroreceptors present in the carotid sinus, aortic arch, and cerebral vessels detect this blood pressure elevation and compensate by signaling the brain. These signals to slow the heart rate and dilate the small blood vessels are received by the brain's vasomotor center by way of the ninth and tenth cranial nerves (glossopharyngeal and vagal).

The vasomotor center responds by reducing the heart rate and decreasing myocardial contractility via impulses from the vagus nerve. At the same time, *efferent impulses* from the spinal cord's sympathetic ganglia dilate the blood vessels above the lesion, causing flushing and sweating.

But the spinal lesion prevents efferent impulses from reaching blood vessels of the lower body below lesion level. As a result, the patient's skin above the lesion appears flushed and hot. Below the lesion, the skin appears pale and is marked by gooseflesh.

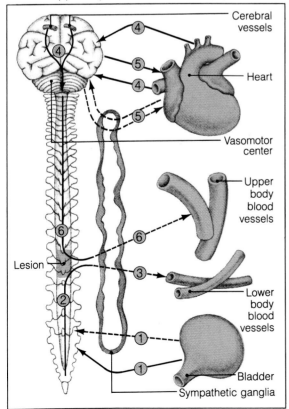

Cerebral vessels

Heart

Vasomotor center

Upper body blood vessels

Lower body blood vessels

Lesion

Bladder

Sympathetic ganglia

How to manage autonomic dysreflexia (AD)

You'll want to be able to understand and recognize AD (hyperreflexia), so you'll be better prepared to care for your patient. Why? Without prompt action to remove the stimulus and decrease the patient's blood pressure, AD may cause seizures, intracranial hemorrhage, and even death.

What causes AD? This complication develops in about 85% of patients with spinal cord lesions at the T_6 level or above. The three most common stimuli include:
• Bladder stimulation from overdistention, either caused by a kinked or blocked catheter, an improperly positioned drainage bag, or urine back-up. Bladder spasms or stones, urinary tract infection, or manual stimulation procedures, such as catheterization and irrigation, may also stimulate the bladder.
• Bowel stimulation from overdistention caused by a fecal impaction, constipation, or excess gas. Other possible stimuli are a rectal exam, manual evacuation, an enema, or suppository insertion.
• Skin stimulation caused by improper turning and positioning, or from treatment manipulation. Autonomic dysreflexia may also be triggered by extreme cold or heat; pressure on the glans penis or testicles; decubitus ulcers; or an ingrown toenail.

Keep in mind that AD may develop suddenly anytime after a spinal injury. Physical reaction to AD is immediate. Its signs and symptoms include: extreme blood pressure elevation; sweating and flushing above the lesion level; chills, gooseflesh, and pale skin below the lesion level; nasal stuffiness; nausea; severe headache; blurred vision; rapid pulse rate which then slows; and metallic taste.

How can AD be managed before it seriously affects your patient? Consider it critical to immediately lower his blood pressure. To do so, elevate the head of his bed to a 45° angle, or help him into a sitting position, unless contraindicated.

Note: Placing a quadriplegic in a sitting position automatically decreases his blood pressure.

Then, notify the doctor. Monitor his blood pressure every 3 to 5 minutes and take immediate action to eliminate the stimulus.

Check to make sure your patient isn't sitting or lying on his catheter, tubing, or drainage bag. Then, check for any obstruction. Palpate his bladder for overdistention. Is his bladder distended? If so, and your patient doesn't have a catheter and can't urinate, gently catheterize him.

Caution: To prevent additional abdominal pressure, never use Credé's maneuver.

If his urine flow is intact and the symptoms persist, check for bowel stimulation. Is your patient impacted? Gently remove the impaction, then apply dibucaine hydrochloride ointment (Nupercainal Ointment*) or lidocaine hydrochloride jelly (Xylocaine Jelly) to his rectum after all the symptoms subside. If he's not impacted, ask him some questions. When was his last bowel movement? Was it hard or soft? Has he had a recent enema? Had a suppository inserted?

If his bladder and bowel are not the sources of the stimulation, check for skin stimulation. Is a sharp object irritating your patient's skin? Have pressure areas developed from leaving him in one position too long? If so, remove the source of pressure or stimulation.

Suppose the symptoms continue to persist 1 to 2 minutes after you've removed the stimulus. Then, you may be ordered by the doctor to administer medications I.V., such as phentolamine methanesulfonate (Regitine), hydralazine hydrochloride (Apresoline*), or diazoxide (Hyperstat*). Continue to monitor your patient's blood pressure 3 to 4 hours after the symptoms subside. Remember, his blood pressure may drop rapidly or AD may recur.

After your patient's condition has stabilized, teach him how to recognize the signs and symptoms of AD. Advise him to contact a doctor immediatey if he feels any of AD's warning signals. Explain to him the importance of a planned bladder and bowel program, and the need for proper body turning and positioning. Remind your patient to periodically check his catheter, tubing, and bag for possible blockage or kinked tubing.

*Available in both the United States and in Canada

Nursing care

Nurses' guide to special beds

When you're caring for a patient with a cervical spine fracture or any other type of neurologic disorder, you'll need to turn and position him every few hours to minimize pressure on his bony prominences. Special beds have been designed to help you do this. These beds help reduce complications, allowing you to turn your patient with less trauma or extraneous movement.

We've detailed four common special beds here. Each one is designed to help you provide the best patient care possible. Based on what your hospital has available, suggest to the doctor which bed you feel will best meet your patient's needs.

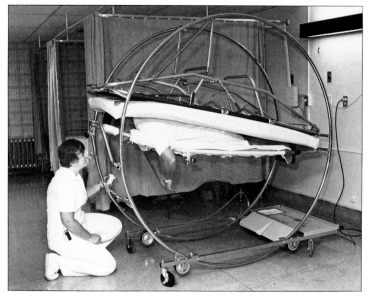

Circle® bed
Description: Rotating bed with two major parts: a bottom mattress and a turning stretcher. A large circular metal frame surrounds your patient.
Functions
* Rotates a full 210°, allowing you to place patient in multiple positions.
* Maintains cervical or pelvic traction when turning.
* A sling that's hooked to the transfer bar provides easy bed-to-wheelchair transfers.
* Can be wheeled to other areas of the hospital with the patient in place.
Nursing considerations
* To minimize nausea and vertigo, don't interrupt the turn until the patient reaches desired position.
* In the event of power failure or motor malfunction, bed may be operated manually.
* Before turning the patient, free any I.V. lines and other equipment so they don't get entangled.
* Maintain eye contact with patient as you turn him.
* If your patient has skull tongs, maintain traction during turn.
* Make sure the equipment is secured to the mobile portion of the frame so it moves easily with him. Take care that the pulley clears the frame during the turn.
* For elimination, secure a bedpan to an opening on the mattress or frame, depending on your patient's position.
* If the patient has copious respiratory drainage, provide a basin to collect secretions.
* When the patient's supine, give him prism glasses to increase his field of vision. With these, he can see all activity at eye level. If he can move his arms, he'll be able to read by holding a book normally rather than having it projected overhead.
* To increase your patient's field of vision, attach a mirror to the upper part of his bed. Remember to remove it before turning him.
* Help patient, as needed, during meals.

* Provide extra padding and skin care on the patient's chin, forehead and back of his head.
* Before turning patient, do the following: check all winged nuts on the head and foot of the bed to make sure they're tight; check his facial mask to make sure patient's eyes and airway are unobstructed; bring the footboard up against his feet; lift the support bar; and position patient's hands around frame, if possible.

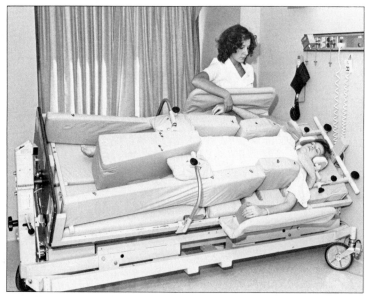

Roto Rest®
Description: Bed is equipped with supportive packs and straps that keep patient's body in proper alignment while gently and continuously rocking him back and forth in a cradle-like fashion.
Functions
* Alleviates need for turning and positioning.
* Maintains patient in relaxed, comfortable position.
* Reduces risk of fecal impaction and constipation, as continuous motion stimulates peristalsis.
* Helps awaken comatose patients by stimulating the vestibular system through constant movement.
* Reduces urinary stasis.
Nursing considerations
* After bathing patient, make sure soap residue is rinsed off his body and the support packs to prevent dermatitis.
* Before turning patient, replace all packs and secure straps.
* Lock bed into extreme lateral position for patient care.
* For elimination, place bedpan under opening in bed.
* Routinely check the patient's knees for signs and symptoms of pressure.
* To avoid disrupting the respiratory system when the head and shoulders assembly is raised, do not tape respiratory tubing to head packs.
* If patient has pulmonary congestion or pneumonia, suction frequently in the first 12 to 24 hours as movement improves drainage and increases secretions.
* Secure any equipment the patient may have, such as I.V. lines or an indwelling (Foley) catheter, to be sure it'll move easily with him.
* When placing patient in a reverse Trendelenburg position, check him frequently to prevent him from moving down in bed or having undue shoulder pressure.
* To help prevent patient isolation and provide stimulation, attach a television to the bed's side.
* Remove foot supporters every 2 hours, as side-to-side motion does not relieve pressure on soles of feet.
* In case of power failure or motor malfunction, turn bed manually and lock in lateral or central position every ½ hour to prevent skin breakdown.

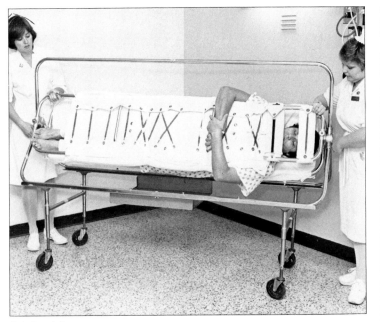

Stryker® frame

Description: An anterior and posterior frame with canvas covers and thin padding over each. The frames, which are supported on a movable cart, have a pivot apparatus at each end.

Functions

● Allows changing a patient's position to either prone or supine by maintaining alignment and immobilization.
● Maintains traction while turning.

Nursing considerations

● To protect your patient's skin, place a foam mattress or padding on both frames before you position him.
● Before turning your patient, secure any equipment he may have, such as an I.V. line, indwelling (Foley) catheter, or respirator tubing to be sure it will not be displaced. Be sure the patient is strapped securely to frame or have him fold his arms around frame, if possible.
● To prevent misalignment, check the equipment periodically and tighten the canvas lacing.
● To aid in maintaining proper alignment, use a footboard, handrolls, bolsters and splints, as required.
● Always remove top frame after turning.
● Turn and position every 2 hours, or more frequently, if indicated.
● You may add armrest wings to the frame at the patient's shoulder level. These will permit him to rest his arms and will help maintain proper alignment.
● For meals, place patient in prone position.
● For elimination, place patient in a supine position, with the bedpan under the opening in the canvas.
● When your patient's prone, monitor him closely for signs of respiratory problems, such as atelectasis and pneumonia. Being in this position may impair his breathing.
● If your patient has skull tongs, maintain traction even when turning. During the turn, have an extra nurse positioned at the patient's head to check pulley and weights.
● Teach your patient how to use the overhead bar to improve the muscle tone in his arms.
● After turning your patient, gently rock frame to be sure it's locked into place.
● To provide some diversion for your patient, move his bed to an outdoor area or recreation room, when possible.
● Never use this bed if your patient: is unable to emotionally adjust to the turning mechanism; can be positioned on his sides; is broader than the external frame; is over 6 feet tall, or over 200 pounds; is unable to assume a safe and comfortable position on the frame because of his physical

structure; is immobilized and hyperextended without the use of skull tongs after a cervical cord injury; or has thoracic or lumbar spine compression fractures reduced by hyperextension.

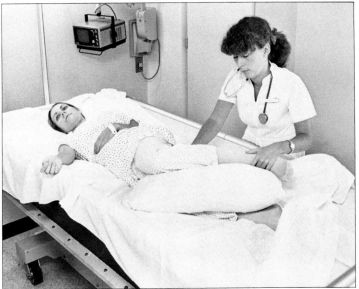

Clinitron®

Description: Air-fluidized support system; a rectangular frame containing 1,800 to 2,000 pounds of silicone-coated glass beads (microspheres) covered with a closely woven monofilament polyester sheet. The beads are fluidized by a flow of warm pressurized air, which floats the polyester cover. The patient is positioned on the cover.

Functions

● Provides a clean, controlled environment.
● Reduces contact pressure.
● Flotation surface temperature can be adjusted to patient's needs.

Nursing considerations

● If a dressing's necessary, keep it as small as possible, as ordered.
● If patient has excessive wound drainage, place a porous dressing under his wound.
● If you use petroleum-based or silver compounds on patient's skin, place an impervious covering over filter sheet. This prevents these compounds from seeping into the microspheres.
● Put a flat sheet over the filter sheet for positioning and transfer.
● If necessary, the patient may be positioned directly on his wound or skin grafts.
● To prevent tears in filter sheet, make sure patient has no pins or clamps on his dressing.
● Check patient frequently for draining plasma, blood, perspiration, and urine. The double-permeable filter sheet allows body fluids to drain into the microspheres and be filtered out.
● Keep patient's room at 75° for maximal system efficiency.
● Select system's temperature according to patient comfort.
● For elimination, roll patient away from you and push the bedpan into the microspheres. Reposition patient on bedpan. Afterward, defluidize the system, and remove the bedpan, by holding it flat as you roll patient away from you with your other hand. Clean patient as usual. Fluidize the system and reposition patient.
● Help patient, as needed, during meals.
● Check to be sure the microspheres are sieved once a month, and between patients.
● Make sure the filter is checked monthly and changed as needed.
● If the microspheres leak onto the floor, wipe up immediately with a damp cloth for safety's sake.
● Check to be sure system's cleaned every week to minimize risk of contamination.

Nursing care

Dealing with daily-care complications

Immobility poses special complication risks. Since the patient with a neurologic injury is usually immobilized or on bed rest, you must be particularly alert for these complications. This chart lists some of the complications of immobility that your patient may experience. It also details the action you can take to prevent or minimize these problems. Don't forget: If you must perform any of these intervention procedures, be sure you explain to the patient beforehand what you're going to do and why. (For details on respiratory complications, see page 141.)

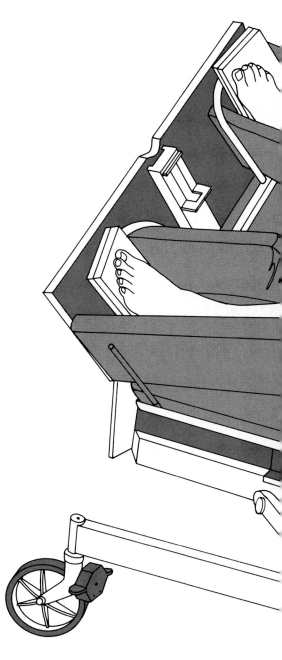

System
Neurologic

Complications
- Dependency
- Disorientation
- Decreased motivation
- Insomnia
- Decreased learning
- Decreased memory
- Apathy
- Withdrawal
- Frustration
- Anger
- Aggression
- Regression

Nursing interventions
- Gradually increase your patient's physical activities. Encourage independency by allowing him to co-manage his care and do as much for himself as possible. Keep him involved and informed on all aspects of his care and therapy.
- Hold frequent conversations with your patient to maintain orientation. Have clocks and calendars in his room. Turn lights off at night.
- Provide your patient with intellectual stimulation. For example, encourage his family to visit, and suggest he read newspapers, books, and magazines, or work crossword puzzles.
- Discourage your patient from taking excessively frequent daytime naps.
- Provide sensory stimulation, such as familiar pictures, ceiling posters, music, or talking books.
- Encourage physical and occupational therapy, as indicated.
- Provide privacy when performing any procedures.
- Spend time with your patient; answer all questions.

System
Integumentary (skin)

Complications
- Painful, reddened areas
- Decubitus ulcers
- Infection

Nursing interventions
- Turn and position your patient regularly, if patient can't do it himself.
- Make sure your patient is on a high-protein, low-calcium diet, with plenty of fluids.
- Observe all skin surfaces, especially bony prominences, for pressure signs, such as blanched or reddened areas. Gently massage reddened areas (especially over bony prominences) to stimulate circulation.
- Keep your patient's skin clean and dry.
- Whenever possible, use a drawsheet or sheepskin to move your patient to avoid irritating his skin.
- When necessary, use special equipment to minimize pressure on your patient's body: an egg crate, air, or water mattress; flotation pads; or heel and elbow protectors.
- Use positioning aids, as needed.
- If the patient does develop a decubitus ulcer, care for it frequently, as ordered.
- If patient has a decubitus ulcer, watch him closely for signs of septicemia, such as increased temperature and purulent drainage. Take cultures, as indicated.
- Administer antibiotics, as ordered.

System
Muscular

Complications
- Contractures
- Decreased muscle tone
- Muscle atrophy

Nursing interventions
- Turn and position your patient regularly, as needed.
- Make sure his body's properly aligned, and that his joints and muscles are well supported.
- Perform range-of-motion (ROM) exercises at least three times a day.
- Use supportive devices, as needed, such as footdrop stops, splints, trochanter rolls, and handrolls.
- When possible, reduce edema by elevating extremities.
- Hyperextend your patient's hips at least three times daily.

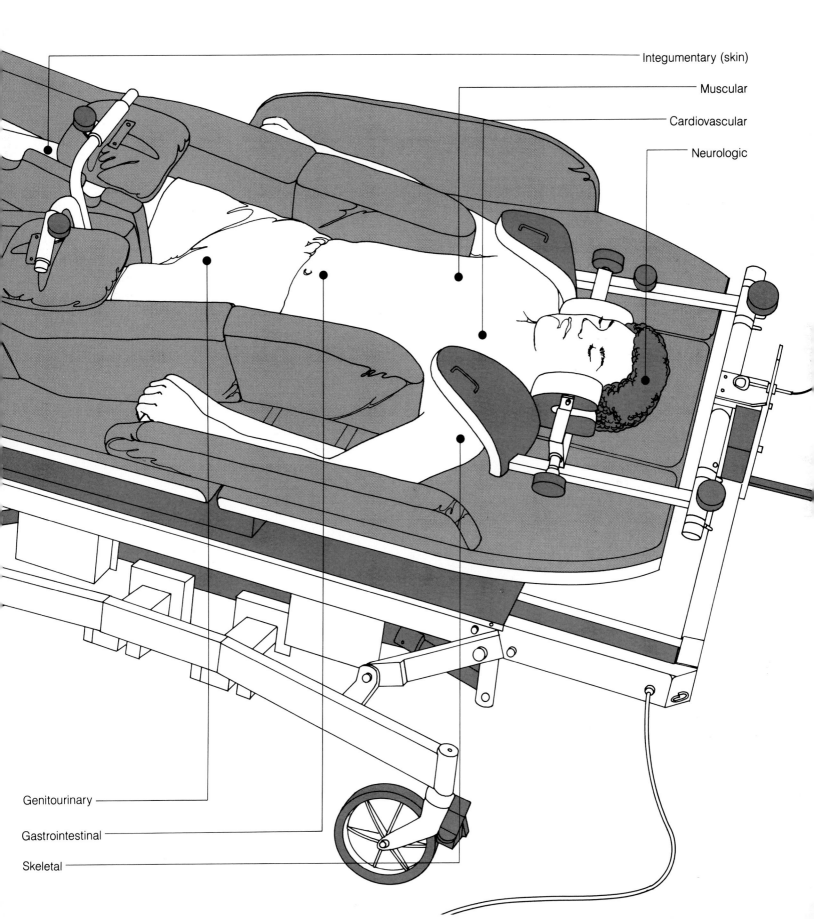

Integumentary (skin)

Muscular

Cardiovascular

Neurologic

Genitourinary

Gastrointestinal

Skeletal

Nursing care

Dealing with daily-care complications continued

System Gastrointestinal	Nursing interventions
Complications • Anorexia • Ileal stasis • Distention • Diarrhea • Constipation • Stress ulcers	• Make sure your patient has a high-roughage, balanced diet, with many of his food preferences. • Arrange for your patient to have several small meals throughout the day instead of three large ones. • Encourage adequate fluid intake; provide your patient with 1,000 to 2,000 ml of fluid daily, unless contraindicated. • Check patient's abdomen every 4 hours for bowel sounds and distention. If distention occurs, measure patient's abdomen every 4 to 8 hours as ordered, and notify the doctor. • Monitor bowel habits. Note amount, color, and consistency of stools. • Check your patient's bowel-movement history. If he's constipated, make sure his medication isn't the cause. • Administer stool softeners, as needed. • For defecation, place your patient in a sitting position, if possible. • Provide privacy for your patient when he's defecating. • As soon as the patient's physical and neurologic condition allows, gradually increase his activities. • Connect nasogastric tube to intermittent, low suction for 24 to 48 hours; then to gravity for 24 hours. • If feeding via nasogastric tube, make sure feedings are easily digestible and high in protein. • If patient can't tolerate feedings, notify doctor. He may order total parenteral nutrition. • Maintain accurate intake and output records. • Observe for signs and symptoms of stress ulcers, especially in patients receiving high doses of corticosteroids. • Administer antacids and cimetidine (Tagamet*) prophylactically, if ordered.

System Genitourinary	Nursing interventions
Complications • Urinary retention • Renal calculi • Urinary tract infections	• Observe your patient's abdomen for bladder distention. If you suspect distention, palpate the area to confirm your findings, and notify the doctor. • Check urine for sediment, which may indicate early formation of renal calculi. If you note any sediment, send a specimen to the lab for analysis. Document the results, and notify the doctor if necessary. • Minimize formation of new renal calculi by acidifying your patient's urine. Make sure he gets adequate amounts of vitamin C. Encourage him to drink orange or cranberry juice, or administer urine acidifiers, as ordered. • Provide at least 1,500 to 2,000 ml of fluids daily, unless contraindicated. • To prevent infection, change indwelling (Foley) catheter routinely; provide catheter care; and avoid irrigations. • Administer urinary tract germicides, such as methenamine mandelate (Mandelamine*), as ordered. • Don't give your patient foods that leave an alkaline ash residue in his urine, such as tomato juice. • When your female patient needs to urinate, place her in a sitting position to allow good urine drainage. If your patient's a male and he's able, have him stand with assistance alongside the bed. Also, provide privacy. • Turn and position patient every 2 hours, or as ordered. • Perform complete range-of-motion (ROM) exercises at least three times a day.

System Skeletal	Nursing interventions
Complications • Backaches • Osteoporosis of disuse (intense pain with weight bearing) • Contractures	• To prevent hip and knee flexion, turn and position your patient regularly, according to his needs. • Make sure his body's properly aligned and that his joints and muscles are well supported. • Help patient perform complete ROM and isometric exercises, as ordered, at least three times a day. Establish a daily program of resistive muscle exercises. • Encourage mobility, and weight bearing, if not contraindicated. Periodically, try to stand your patient upright so he bears his weight, or use a tilt table. • Be sure footboards are used properly. Place your patient's feet flat against the footboard so they form a 90° angle to his legs. • Be sure patient's mattress is firm. Use a bedboard if necessary. • Make sure your patient gets a high-protein, low-calcium diet with plenty of fluids. • Check his urine for sediment, which may indicate early formation of renal calculi. If you note any sediment, send a urine specimen to the lab for analysis. Document the results and notify the doctor, if necessary. • To prevent constipation, provide a high-roughage diet; administer stool softeners; give plenty of fluids; establish good bowel routine; and be sure patient's well supported in sitting position during defecation, if possible.

System Cardiovascular	Nursing interventions
Complications • Decreased myocardial tone • Venous stasis • Thrombus formation • Orthostatic hypotension	• To alleviate signs and symptoms of orthostatic hypotension, gradually elevate head of bed to sitting position, dangle his legs over side of bed prior to chair sitting, and stand patient before placing him in chair. • To prevent increased workload on the patient's heart, instruct him how to turn with minimal effort, use overhead frame with trapeze bar, and take deep, slow breaths while turning. • Gradually increase your patient's activities to avoid fatigue. • Apply antiembolism stockings, as ordered. Remove them at least once every 24 hours. • Elevate legs at hips rather than knees. Keep legs elevated above heart level. • Place a pillow between patient's legs while he's on his side. Keep his upper leg positioned more anteriorly than his lower leg. • Encourage foot and leg exercises. • Make sure your patient has a high-protein, low-calcium diet, with plenty of fluids. • Instruct your patient to exhale slowly when moving in bed to prevent him from performing a Valsalva maneuver.

*Available in both the United States and in Canada

Learning about exercise programs

Regardless of your patient's neurologic disorder, you'll be responsible for helping plan and implement an exercise program tailored to his condition and needs. An effective exercise program, performed at least three times a day, will help your patient function at maximum capacity during his hospital stay, and at home.

When we talk about an exercise program, we're referring to range-of-motion (ROM) exercises that take your patient's joints through their full extent of movement. These exercises also maintain joint activity, stimulate blood circulation, and promote muscle tone.

Where do you begin? First, you'll need to check your patient's care plan, medical history, physical condition, and emotional status. Consult with your patient's doctor and physical therapist. Depending on your hospital's policy, they may select your patient's ROM exercise program, or instruct you to do so.

The three basic types of ROM programs are:
• Active: helps strengthen weakened joints and is performed by the patient. For more information and a home care aid on this program, see pages 127 to 131.
• Active-assistive: helps strengthen and maintain joint activity and motion. The patient performs these exercises with minimal assistance from another person.
• Passive: maintains joint activity and motion. These exercises are performed for the patient by another person; for example, a nurse or family member.

Before beginning your patient's exercise program, explain its importance to your patient and his family. Answer any questions they may have. Encourage the patient to be as active as physically possible. Also take this opportunity to encourage the family to take part in the patient's exercise program. Besides physically helping the patient (if needed), remind them that they play an important part in supporting and encouraging the patient. Then, show the patient and his family the complete program. (For more details on ROM programs, see the NURSING PHOTOBOOK PROVIDING EARLY MOBILITY.)

Document the procedure, program selected, and any patient teaching, in your nurses' notes.

Coping with your patient's emotional needs

Caring for a patient with a neurologic disorder requires tremendous amounts of time, patience, and energy. Not only will you have to deal with your patient's physical condition, you'll also need to help your patient and his family adjust emotionally.

Sound difficult? It doesn't have to be. But first, you'll have to assess your feelings and emotions. Know your limitations. You'll need to be able to accept your patient's condition realistically, yet with a positive attitude. Remember, if you have difficulty dealing with a patient, ask a co-worker to take over for you. Any uneasiness or irritation you feel will be projected to your patient and his family.

When you enter your patient's room, always greet him first. If he wants to talk, sit down and chat with him for several minutes.

Reinforce your verbal messages by touching his hand. Or, if he doesn't have sensation in his hand, touch his forehead. Then, attend to any special equipment he may have. Keep in mind that equipment is only a tool in nursing. It can't replace the attention and care you should give your patient and his family.

As you probably know, a patient's reaction to his neurologic disorder will vary from individual to individual. He may feel:
• Anger: *I hate you and everybody in this hospital!*
• Fear: *I'll never be able to enjoy life again.*
• Denial: *In a couple of weeks, I'll be fine; this setback is only temporary.*
• Acceptance: *I'm going to live my life to its fullest.*

Try to understand the effect your patient's condition has on his and his family's emotions. Don't hesitate to share your feelings and emotions with your patient and his family. Let them know you're human.

Remember: Sharing your patient's feelings and concerns will help build a rapport with him.

However, in addition to adjusting to his condition, the patient, his family—and you—may also have to cope with unpredictable setbacks whenever they occur; for example respiratory infections and emergency surgery. Try to help your patient and his family deal with these crises. Be supportive and understanding.

Now, here are some important guidelines to remember whenever you care for a patient with a neurologic disorder:
• Explain your patient's disorder, and any procedures that may be necessary, to him and his family. Doing so will help them know what to expect.
• Try to find out what your patient and his family know about his disorder.
• Clear up any misconceptions. For example, is the patient afraid he'll never be able to return home?
• Find out how your patient and his family feel about his disorder. For example, does the patient resent his dependency, lack of privacy, and hospital restriction on visitors? If possible, ask the doctor to relax some of the visiting restrictions.
• Talk to your patient and his family and encourage them to express their feelings of denial, anger, and fear.
• Help the patient and his family understand any special equipment he may have, such as I.V. lines, an indwelling (Foley) catheter, an artificial respirator, or a cardiac monitor.
• Encourage your patient to be as self-sufficient as possible. Praise him for his efforts.

And finally, document all patient teaching, and your patient's reaction to it, in your nurses' notes. That way, the next nurse on duty can build on your foundation.

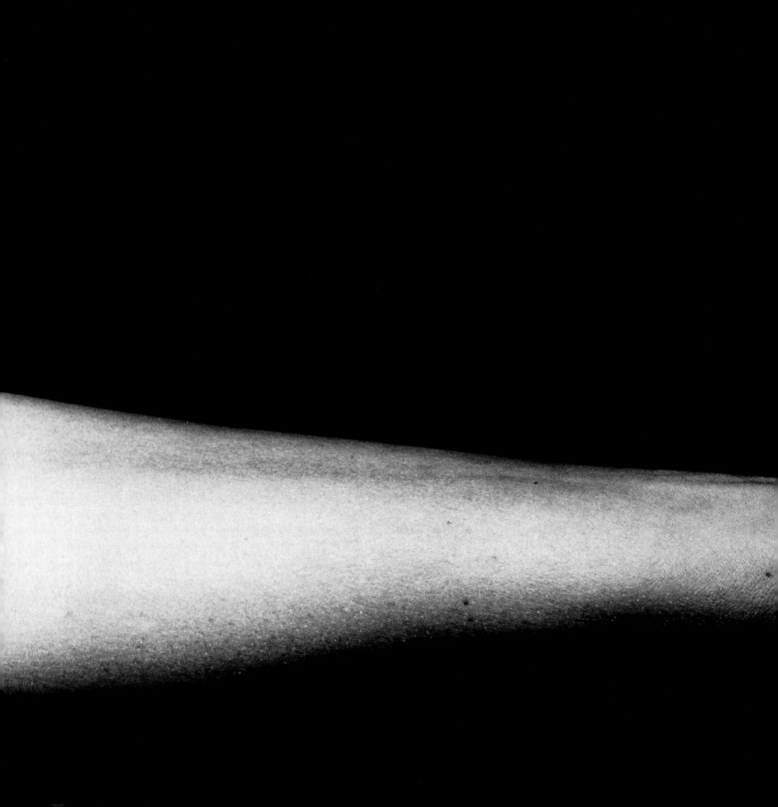

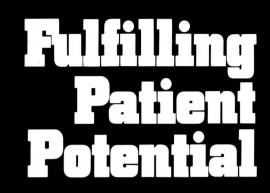

Fulfilling Patient Potential

Positioning and exercise
Respiratory function
Bowel and bladder function
Sexual function

Positioning and exercise

For the patient with a neurologic disorder, leaving the hospital may be overwhelming. Your patient will need to readjust to home surroundings, while continuing to develop physically and emotionally to his maximum potential.

How can you help? Make your patient's rehabilitation an ongoing process from the moment he enters your unit. Then, teach your patient and his family how to continue his rehabilitation program at home. Show them positioning and exercise basics, and tell them how to cope with any problems that they may encounter.

In the pages that follow, we'll prepare you for this special challenge. We'll show you how to help your patient and his family:
• set realistic goals.
• apply antiembolism stockings.
• perform a stand-pivot transfer.

In addition, you'll find a home care aid reviewing active range-of-motion exercises, and step-by-step instructions for using a transfer board. Read these pages carefully.

Placing your patient in a supine position

1 *You're caring for Jena Montgomery, a 43-year-old real estate broker with right hemiparesis as the result of a brain lesion. To help prepare her for discharge, you'll need to teach positioning and turning basics to Mrs. Montgomery and her family. Do you know how? Follow these steps carefully.*
Begin by explaining to them how the proper positioning and exercising can help prevent contractures and decubitus ulcers. Familiarize Mrs. Montgomery and her family with a positioning schedule. Be sure to emphasize that Mrs. Montgomery should be turned every 2 hours, and that the positioning schedule must be followed.
Then, check to be sure the bed is level with your waist, and flat. Lower the right side rail. Tell the family that lowering the side rail provides easy patient access.

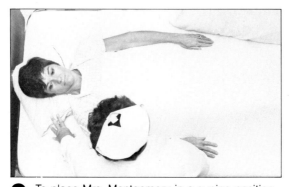

2 To place Mrs. Montgomery in a supine position, put a small pillow diagonally under her head, as the nurse is doing here. Remember, more than one pillow, or a large, bulky one, may obstruct her airway or cause contractures. Then, align Mrs. Montgomery's head with her spine. Make sure she's positioned so she's looking at the ceiling.

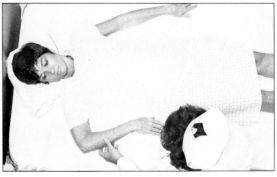

3 Next, position Mrs. Montgomery's arms at her sides, palms down. Then, to minimize dependent edema in her affected side, place a pillow under her right arm, aligning it from the shoulder joint to beyond her fingers. Slightly bend her right elbow and point it away from her trunk, as the nurse is doing in this photo.

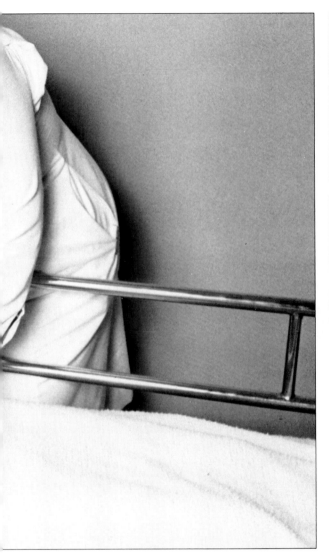

5 To position Mrs. Montgomery's trunk and legs, check to make sure her back is flat on the bed. Fold a small towel and place it at the small of her back for additional support.

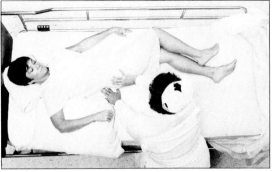

6 Point her knees and toes toward the ceiling. Elevate her right leg with one pillow, aligning it just below the hip joint to the calf.

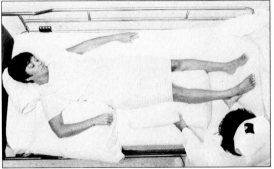

7 Now, roll a small towel and place it under Mrs. Montgomery's right ankle, as shown. This will prevent pressure on her right heel.

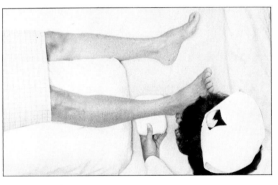

8 Tuck the edge of a large towel or blanket under her right hip, as shown, and roll it inward until the towel is pressed firmly against her thigh. Doing so prevents abduction of all lower joints which could lead to deformities or contractures. Put up the side rail.
Document the procedure in your nurses' notes.

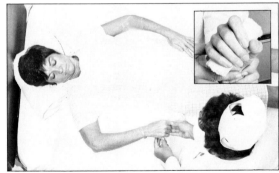
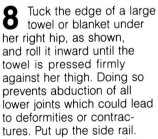

4 Now, fold a small washcloth or towel lengthwise. Roll it as shown here. Place the rolled cloth in Mrs. Montgomery's affected hand, as shown. To avoid excessive pressure or further injury, check that her thumb is in opposition to her fingers and that her four fingers cover the entire cloth roll.

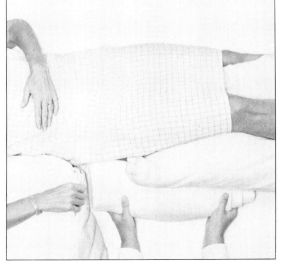

Positioning and exercise

How to position your patient laying on her side

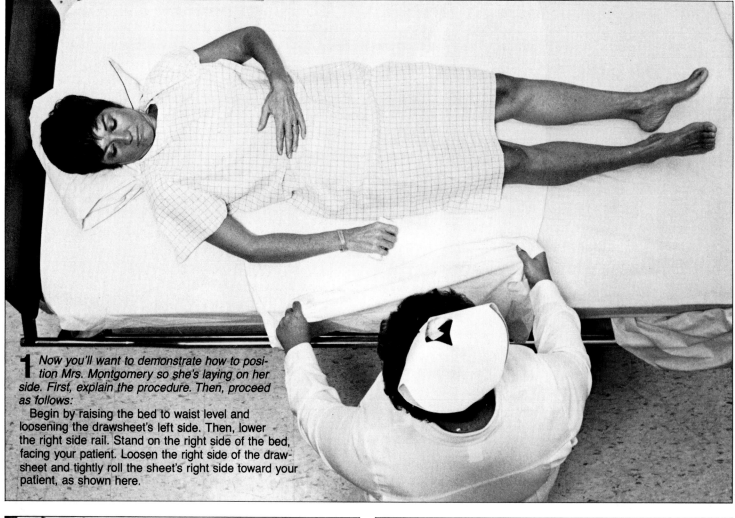

1 *Now you'll want to demonstrate how to position Mrs. Montgomery so she's laying on her side. First, explain the procedure. Then, proceed as follows:*
Begin by raising the bed to waist level and loosening the drawsheet's left side. Then, lower the right side rail. Stand on the right side of the bed, facing your patient. Loosen the right side of the drawsheet and tightly roll the sheet's right side toward your patient, as shown here.

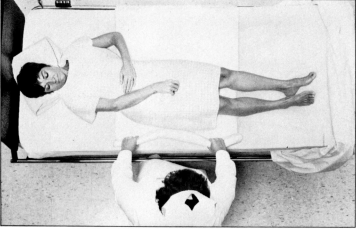

2 Now, firmly grasp the sheet's rolled end with both hands, placing one hand near Mrs. Montgomery's hip and the other near her knee. Gently pull the sheet and your patient toward you, as the nurse is doing here. Then, align her body.

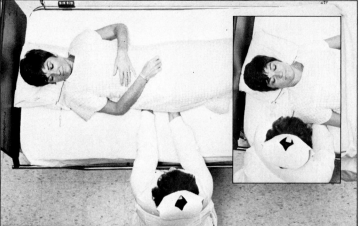

3 What if you don't have a drawsheet? Slide your hands (palms up) under Mrs. Montgomery's hips. Pull her lower body and legs toward you.
[Inset] Then, slide your hands (palms up) under Mrs. Montgomery's shoulders. Pull her shoulders and upper body toward you.

4 Raise the right side rail. Move to the left side of the bed and lower the left side rail. Face Mrs. Montgomery. Bring her right arm across her chest, as shown here, and make sure her left arm's abducted.
Important: Bend your patient's right knee, and cross her right leg over her left before continuing.

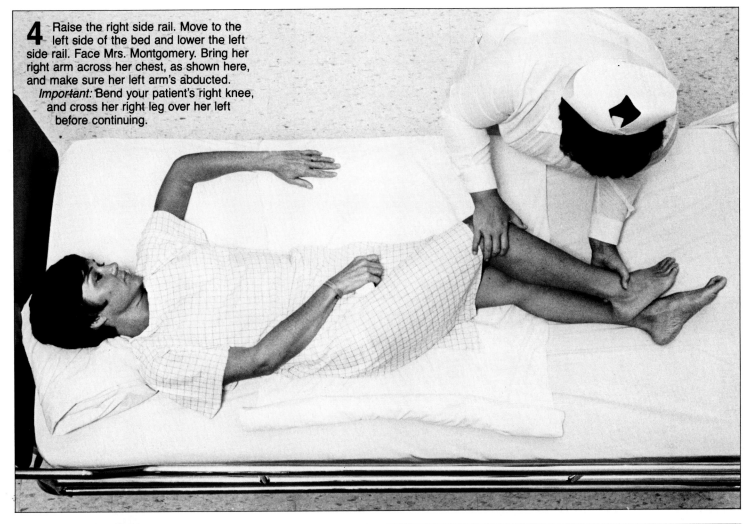

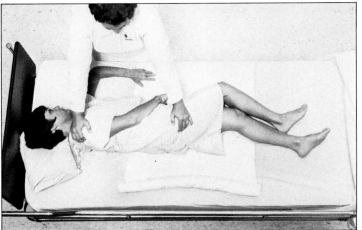

5 Place your right hand on Mrs. Montgomery's right shoulder. Position your left hand on her right hip. Pulling with both hands simultaneously, roll her onto her left side, as shown.

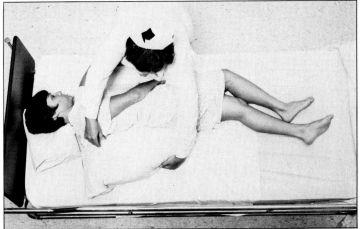

6 Now, tuck a pillow lengthwise behind Mrs. Montgomery, from her shoulder to her coccyx. Make sure the pillow fits snugly against her back.

Positioning and exercise

How to position your patient laying on her side continued

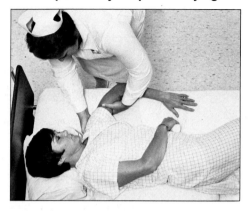

7 Reposition a pillow under her head and neck, as shown.
Gently pull your patient's left shoulder toward you. Make sure her arm is abducted at approximately a 45° angle to the rest of her body.

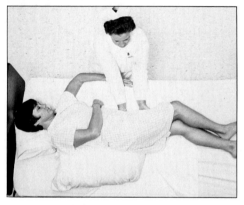

8 Next, flex her left elbow at a 90° angle, and turn her left palm down.
Gently pull your patient's left hip toward you.

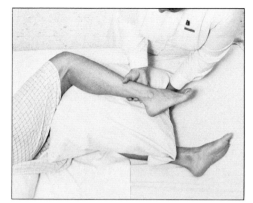

9 Now, place a large pillow lengthwise under her right leg and foot, from knee to ankle, as shown. Keep her lower leg flat and extended. Always keep a pillow between Mrs. Montgomery's right and left legs. Doing so prevents pressure sores.

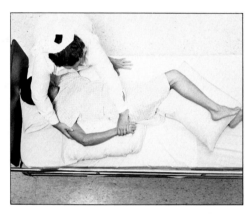

10 Place Mrs. Montgomery's right elbow on a pillow. Extend her right arm away from her body, slightly bending it at the right elbow, as shown.

11 Or have Mrs. Montgomery grasp a pillow with both arms. Lay her right arm on the pillow, palm down if possible.
Raise the right side rail. To position your patient on her right side, follow the same steps, reversing the directions.
Be sure to document all positioning changes in your nurses' notes and on the patient's chart.

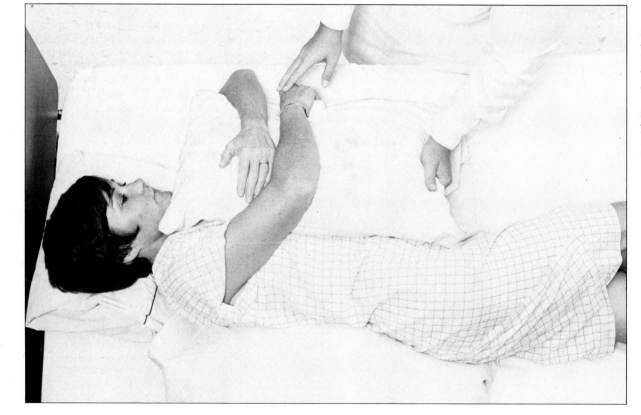

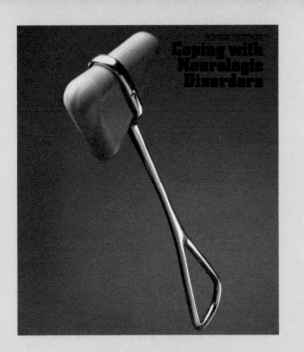

This is your order card. Send no money.

Discover how easily this introductory PHOTOBOOK, *Coping with Neurologic Disorders,* can improve your nursing skills. Close-up photographs and concise captions show you step by step how to:

- test and assess cranial nerves
- prepare your patient for CT scan
- perform a neuro check
- manage spinal cord injuries
- help your patient fulfill his potential.

Here's all you need to know to care effectively for the patient with neurologic problems. So send for your 10-day, free examination of this important new PHOTOBOOK today.

© 1982 Intermed Communications, Inc.

10-DAY FREE TRIAL

USE THE CARD ABOVE TO:

1. **Subscribe to the NURSING PHOTOBOOK™ series (and save $1.00 on each book you buy)**

   or

2. **Buy *Coping with Neurologic Disorders* without joining the series (and pay only $13.95 for your copy)**

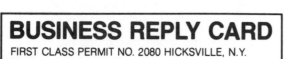
Introduce yourself to the brand-new NURSING PHOTOBOOK™ series

…the remarkable breakthrough in nursing education that can change your career. Each book in this unique series contains detailed *Photostories*… and tables, charts, and graphs to help you learn important new procedures. And each handsome PHOTOBOOK offers you • 160 illustrated, fact-filled pages • brilliant, high-contrast photographs • convenient 9"x10½" size • durable, hardcover binding • carefully chosen bibliography • complete index. Watch the experts at work showing you how to… administer drugs… teach your patient about his illness and its treatment… minimize trauma… understand doctors' diagnoses… increase patient comfort… and much more. Discover how you can become a better nurse by joining this exciting new series. You can examine each PHOTOBOOK at your leisure… for 10 days *absolutely free!*

Be sure to mail the postage-paid card at left to reserve *your* first copy of *Nursing82.*

Nursing82 gives you clear, concise instruction in "hands-on" nursing. Every issue brings you in-depth clinical articles about the newest developments in nursing care—what's being discovered, researched, treated, cured. You'll learn about the new procedures, new techniques, new medications, and new equipment that will mean more skills and knowledge for you…better care for your patients!

Order *your* subscription today!

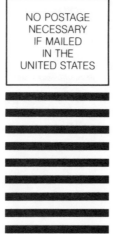

How to place your patient in a prone position

1 *You are now ready to change Mrs. Montgomery's position from laying on her side to laying on her abdomen (prone position). Tell her what you plan to do and remind her to keep clutching the handroll. Note: Prone position may be contraindicated for some patients, such as those with respiratory distress, or loss of consciousness.*

First, raise Mrs. Montgomery's bed to a level slightly below your waist, and lower the right side rail. Move her to the right side of the bed, and remove any pillows or other supportive devices. Turn her head so that her cheek is on the bed. Raise the right side rail.

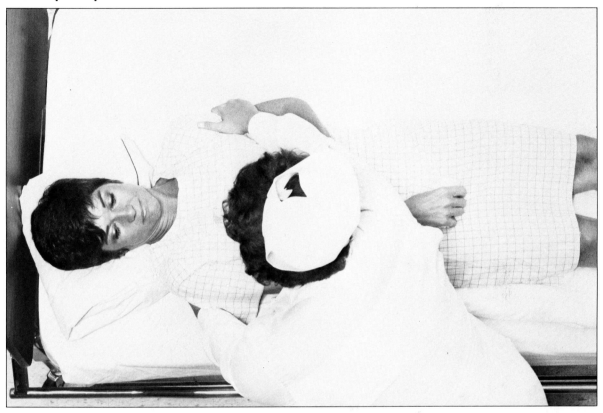

2 Move to the left side of the bed. Lower the left side rail. Now, straighten Mrs. Montgomery's left arm gently. Position it, palm up, next to her left side.

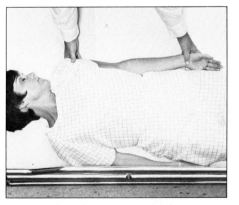

3 Tuck her left palm under her left thigh, as the nurse is doing in this photo.

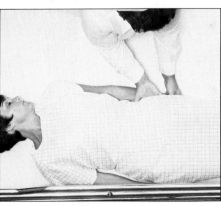

4 Flex her right leg at the hip and knee. Position her right arm so it rests on her body.

Place your right hand on her right shoulder and your left hand on Mrs. Montgomery's right hip.

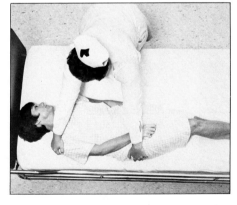

5 Slowly roll Mrs. Montgomery toward you onto her abdomen. Make sure her left arm's not under her and that her airway's unobstructed.

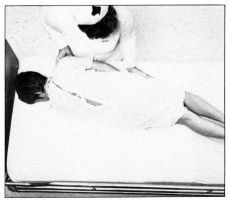

Positioning and exercise

How to place your patient in a prone position continued

6 Carefully position her right arm, as the nurse is doing here. Now, roll a small towel and position it under her right shoulder. Check to be sure her right shoulder is completely off the bed. If it isn't, reposition the towel.

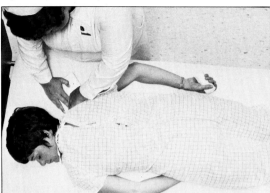

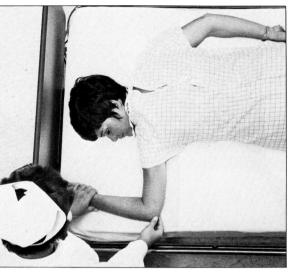

7 Then, carefully abduct her left arm, placing it at a 90° angle to her body. Flex her left elbow up, positioning her forearm at a 90° angle to her upper arm.
   Roll a small towel and place it under her left shoulder, as shown here.
   Make sure Mrs. Montgomery is still clutching the handroll in her right hand.

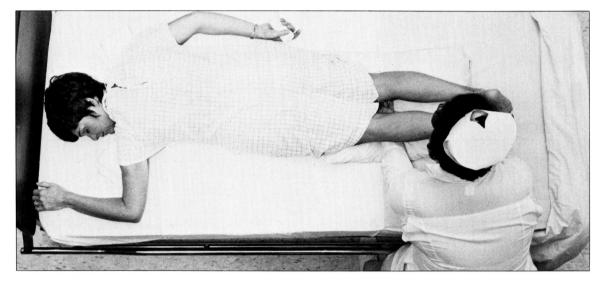

8 Next, position a large pillow lengthwise under her legs, from her knees to her ankles.

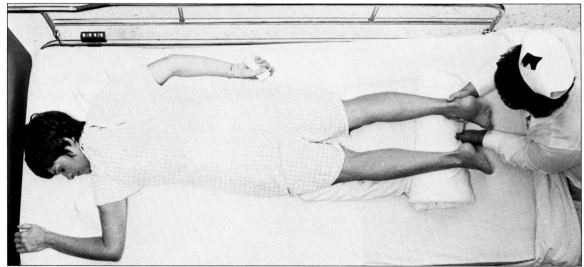

9 Then, roll a large towel and place it perpendicular to the pillow under both ankles, as shown. Check to be sure both feet are suspended between the towel and the end of the bed. To make her more comfortable, place a small pillow under her head. Pull up the left side rail.
   Document the position change in your notes and on your patient's positioning chart.

Establishing a positioning and skin-care schedule

Of course you know how important maintaining a turning, positioning, and skin-care schedule is for your patient. Not only does such a schedule help prevent decubitus ulcers and contractures, but it may also prevent respiratory, circulatory, genitourinary, and gastrointestinal complications. But how can you stress the importance of a turning, positioning, and skin-care schedule to the patient and his family?

For starters, set up a mutually agreeable time to talk with the patient and his family about the schedule. Explain that you'll need their assistance to help devise a schedule tailored to their needs. Then, carefully assess both the patient's condition and his day-to-day activities, as well as those of the family. Here are some guidelines to review with the family:
• Try to plan position changes and skin care around your patient's activities. Encourage him to participate as much as possible in developing the schedule. For example, does he want to be laying on his side when he receives visitors?

How to help your patient set goals

Twenty-six-year-old Paul Bindell, a professional baseball player, is admitted to your unit with newly diagnosed Huntington's chorea. He's apprehensive and says his life is over. Not only is he afraid he'll lose his job and that he'll never be able to function as the head of his household, he's also worried he'll never function sexually. He's unsure of his ability to financially support his wife and 3-month-old son, Jeremy. He's scared he may have passed the disease on to Jeremy. Mrs. Bindell is also affected. She's naturally worried about her husband and son and is overwhelmed by the responsibility she suddenly has to assume.

As a nurse, you play an important role in helping the couple adjust to Mr. Bindell's condition. Where do you begin? For starters, assess your knowledge and feelings. You'll need to accept your patient's condition realistically, yet with a positive attitude. Maintain control over your emotions and learn all the facts about Huntington's chorea. Investigate the disease and its process. As soon as possible, encourage the couple to talk with you about Mr. Bindell's condition, and their feelings. Clear up any misconceptions they may have. Answer their questions completely and honestly.

If the Bindells tell you they're not ready to talk, give them some time to adjust. But, keep the lines of communication open.

As you perform Mr. Bindell's daily care, try to develop a good rapport with him. You'll need to gain his confidence and cooperation.

Then, try to set up a mutually agreeable time to talk with Mr. Bindell about his future goals. If he seems agitated, fatigued, or depressed, postpone your discussion to another time. Then,

• Ask the doctor whether any of the positions or positioning aids you've chosen may be contraindicated.
• Use your common sense. Some patients may need to be turned more often than at the normal 2 or 3 hour intervals. Tell the family to look for blanched or reddened areas on the patient's skin. If they see any, advise them to massage them, turn him immediately, and adjust his schedule.
• Document the positioning schedule on the patient's care plan, and keep a copy at his bedside. Doing so allows others to know when he was last turned.
• Revise the schedule as the patient's physical and mental condition improves or deteriorates.
• Observe each position's effectiveness. Note whether joint motion is being decreased, maintained, or increased.

Remember, a good schedule always takes into consideration the patient's activities and how he feels. Develop your plan accordingly.

when he's ready to talk, suggest including his wife and family.

During your goal-setting session, encourage Mr. Bindell to set some long-term goals that are attainable and realistic. Be sure he understands that all goals should reflect his own capabilities and not represent the possibly unrealistic goals of his family, friends, or hospital staff members.

Keep in mind that Mr. Bindell will probably find it easier to set short-term goals. By achieving these goals, he'll be able to see progress in a short time. Doing so may help alleviate some of his frustration and impatience. Later, after he gains confidence, he may be able to work toward setting long-term goals. Remember, short-term goals should be easily attainable. Some possible short-term goals for your patient may be:
• brushing his teeth
• feeding himself
• washing his face.

A possible long-term goal for Mr. Bindell may be performing all activities of daily living within his physical and functional capabilities.

Important: Never set inflexible time limits for short-term or long-term goals. As you know, each patient will achieve his goals at his own speed.

You'll also want to familiarize the Bindells with various outside agencies that will keep the patient's progress ongoing; for example: genetic counseling, vocational training, social services, and the visiting nurses association. If they seem receptive, contact the agencies for them.

And finally, always praise your patient for his participation in the goal-setting session.

Positioning and exercise

Home care

How to strengthen your muscles and joints

Dear Patient:
Now that you're ready to return home, you'll need to continue strengthening and toning your muscles. By exercising twice a day, you'll find it easier to carry out your day-to-day activities. Repeat each exercise five times on the muscle or joint being strengthened. *Important:* If you feel severe pain when performing any of these exercises, stop immediately. If pain persists, notify your doctor. Never force or overstretch a muscle, as you may cause further damage.

And remember, to get maximum benefit out of this program, perform each exercise slowly and gently. Try performing all the exercises the nurse has circled on these sheets in the morning, and again before dinner. Work the exercises into your daily routine; for example, exercise as you bathe, or while sitting in a chair watching T.V.

Note: If you're performing the exercises in a bed or chair with wheels, make sure they're locked before you begin.

Use these instructions as a guide:

1 **Neck exercises:** Keeping your shoulders level, touch your chin to your right shoulder, or as close to it as possible. Then, touch your chin to your left shoulder or as close to it as possible. Do not raise your shoulder to your chin. Return to the starting position.

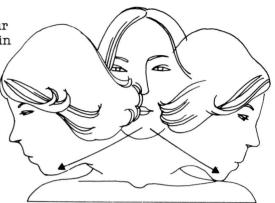

2

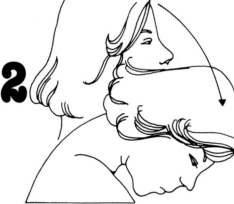

Now, touch your chin to your chest, or as close to it as possible. Raise your chin to starting position.

3 Next, bend your head and neck backward, as far as possible. Return your head to starting position.

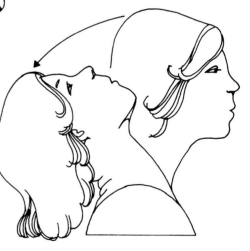

Rotate your head and neck clockwise. Then, rotate your head and neck counterclockwise.

4

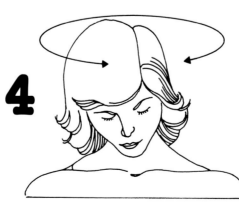

1 **Trunk exercises:** Sit on a chair so your legs are straight and your arms hang loosely at your side. Bend forward as far as possible. Return to starting position.

2 Now, maintaining the same position, bend to the right side, making sure you bend from the waist. Then, bend to the left. Return to starting position.

3 Next, stand with your feet 2″ (5.1 cm) apart. Let your arms hang loosely at your sides—and without bending your knees—bend backward, as far as possible. Return to starting position.

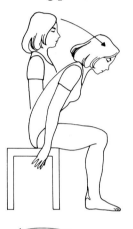

4 Keeping your hips facing straight ahead, twist your upper body to the right as far as possible. Then, twist your body to the left as far as possible. Return to starting position.

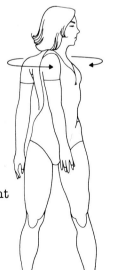

1 **Shoulder exercises:** Standing straight with your arms at your sides, raise your right arm forward and upward (over your head), as far as possible. Return to starting position, and repeat the exercise with your left arm.

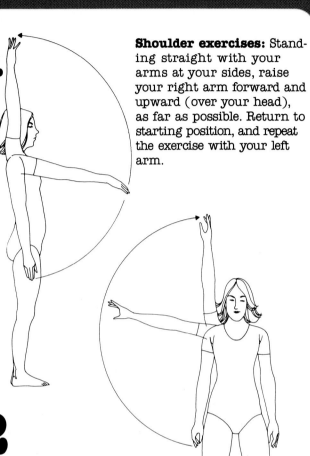

2 Now, standing with your arms at your sides, raise your right arm sideways and upward, over your head, or as far as possible. Return your right arm to starting position and repeat the exercise with your left arm.

3 Maintaining the same position, raise your right arm to shoulder level. Then bring your arm across your body toward your left shoulder, or as close to it as possible. Return your arm to starting position, and repeat the exercise with your left arm.

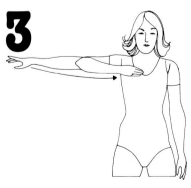

Positioning and exercise

Home care

How to strengthen your muscles and joints continued

1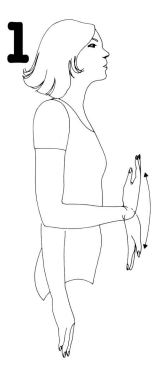

Wrist exercises:
Keeping your upper right arm at your side, bend your elbow so your forearm is at a 90° angle to your upper arm. Turn your palm up so it's facing the ceiling. Now, without bending your elbow, raise your hand as far as possible. Then, lower your hand as far as possible. Return your hand to starting position, and repeat the exercise with your left hand.

2 Next, maintaining the same position, move your hand toward your body as close to it as possible. Then move your hand away from your body, as far from it as possible. Return to starting position and repeat the exercise with your left hand.

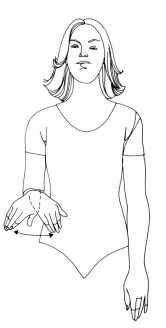

1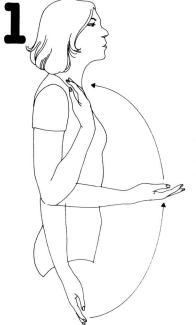

Elbow exercises:
For this exercise, you can sit in a chair, or stand, whichever is most comfortable. Let your arms hang loosely at your side. Then, bending your right elbow, bring your fingertips to your right shoulder, or as close to it as possible. Return your right arm to starting position and repeat the exercise with your left arm.

1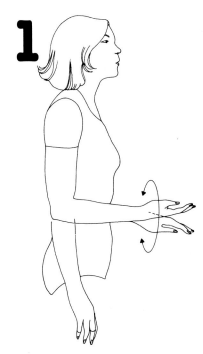

Forearm exercises:
Keeping your upper right arm at your side, bend your elbow so your forearm's at a 90° angle to your upper arm and your palm is facing the ceiling. Turn your palm down, then up. Repeat the exercise with your left hand.

1 **Knee exercises:** For this exercise, you can sit on the bed with your legs straight ahead of you or lie on your abdomen with your legs extended. Bend your right knee as much as possible. Return to starting position, and repeat the exercise with your left knee.

1 **Hip exercises:** Now, lie on your back and bend your right knee. Bring your knee toward your chest, or as close to it as possible. Return your knee to starting position, and repeat the exercise with your left knee.

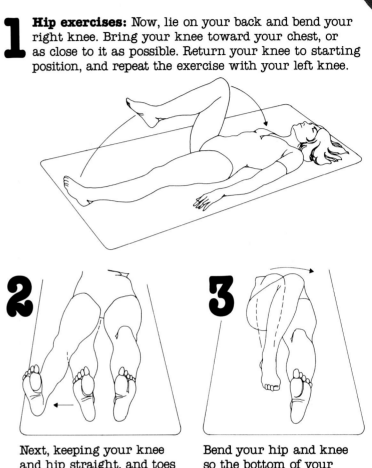

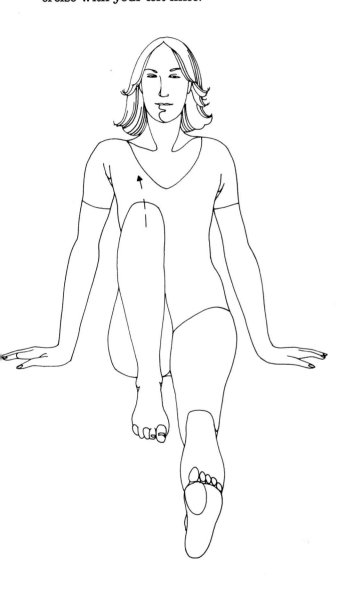

2 Next, keeping your knee and hip straight, and toes pointed upwards, move your right leg to the right as far as possible. Return to starting position and repeat the exercise with your left leg.

3 Bend your hip and knee so the bottom of your right foot is flat on the bed. Roll your leg inward as far as possible. Return to starting position, and repeat the exercise with the left leg.

4 Now, maintaining the same position with your back and hips flat on the bed, raise your right leg upward as far as possible. Return your right leg to starting position and repeat the exercise with your left leg.

Positioning and exercise

Using a Trans-Aid® institutional lifter to move your patient from a bed to a wheelchair

1 *Thirty-six-year-old Tyler Graham is a paraplegic. Because he's unable to transfer himself, you use a mechanical lifter. Now, you want to show Mr. Graham's family how to use this equipment so they'll be prepared for his return home. Follow these guidelines carefully.*

Note: In this photostory, the nurse is using a Trans-Aid™ institutional lifter and sling.

Place a wheelchair to the left of the bed, leaving enough room to operate the lifter. Lock the chair's wheels and move the legrests out of the way.

Then, explain the procedure to your patient and reassure him. Also explain the procedure to his family.

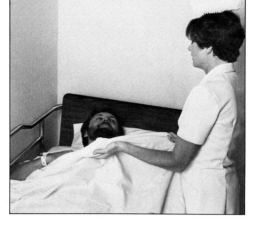

2 Now, roll Mr. Graham onto his right side. Fanfold the sling, and place it behind him. Position all hooks with the open ends away from his body. Make sure the white hooks are next to his right shoulder and the gold hooks are behind his right knee.

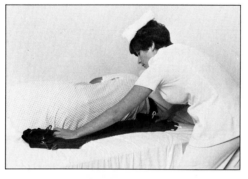

3 Roll your patient onto his left side as you unfold the sling. Then, place him in a supine position in the center of the sling with his body well-aligned.

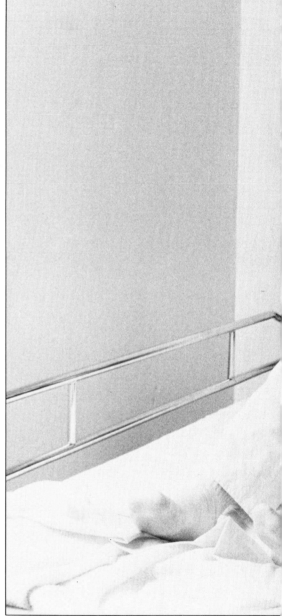

4 Now you're ready to position the lifter above your patient, as the nurse is doing in this photo.

Attach the white hooks to the silver chain and the gold hooks to the gold chain.

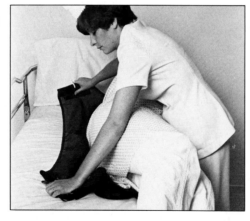

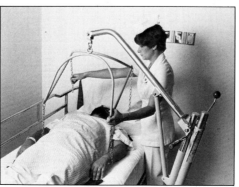

5 Firmly turn the handle of the lifter clockwise to raise Mr. Graham to a sitting position. Then, stop turning and check to be sure he's positioned properly. If he's not, lower him to the bed by turning the handle counterclockwise. Reposition the sling. If everything's okay, continue to raise the sling until Mr. Graham's suspended just above the bed. Keep your arm under your patient's knees during the procedure to guide him.

[Inset] Now, slowly turn the sling so your patient's legs hang over the edge of the bed.

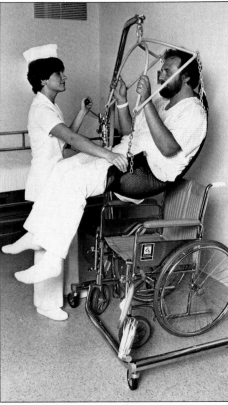

6 Move the lifter toward the wheelchair. Now, position him directly above the wheelchair's seat.

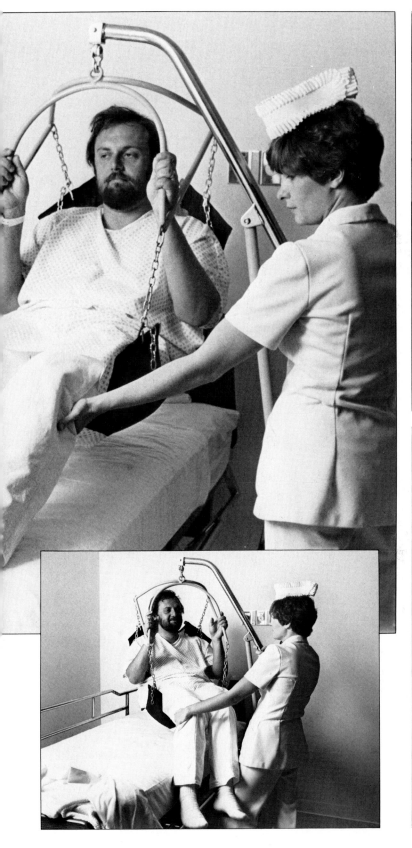

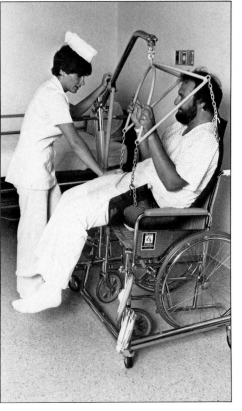

7 Slowly turn the lifter's handle counterclockwise to lower Mr. Graham into the seat. When the chains become slack, stop turning.

Unhook the sling from the lifter. Leave the sling under your patient. To prevent skin irritation, smooth any folds you see in the sling. Then, position your patient properly in the chair.

Document the procedure and family teaching in your nurses' notes. When it's time to move Mr. Graham back to bed, have a family member assist with the procedure.

Positioning and exercise

Teaching your patient how to use a transfer board

1 *Consider this: Jordan Stafford, a 36-year-old building inspector, has a spinal cord transection. As a result, he's paralyzed from the waist down. Up to this point, you've been assisting Mr. Stafford into a wheelchair by using a mechanical lifter. But now, the doctor feels Mr. Stafford's strong enough to move himself from bed to wheelchair using the transfer board, and asks you to teach Mr. Stafford this procedure. Do you know how? Follow these steps:*

First, explain the procedure to Mr. Stafford and assure him you'll help if necessary. Then, make sure his wheelchair has removable armrests and legrests. Position his wheelchair next to the bed so the right side of the chair is next to the left side of the bed. Have him lock the chair's wheels in place (see inset).

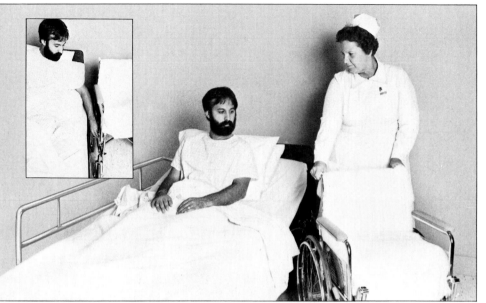

2 Show Mr. Stafford how to remove the wheelchair's legrests. Then, adjust his bed, so it's level with the wheelchair seat (left photo). Now have Mr. Stafford remove the wheelchair's left armrest and hang it from the wheelchair handles (right photo).

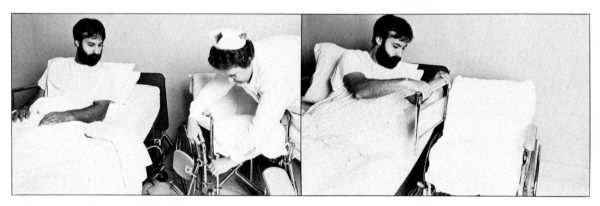

3 Now, instruct Mr. Stafford to shift his weight onto his right buttock. Help him slide the transfer board under his buttocks and upper thighs.

[Inset] Have him extend the other end of the board onto the wheelchair.

Before he begins his transfer, remind Mr. Stafford to check to make sure the board is resting securely on the wheelchair seat and the bed.

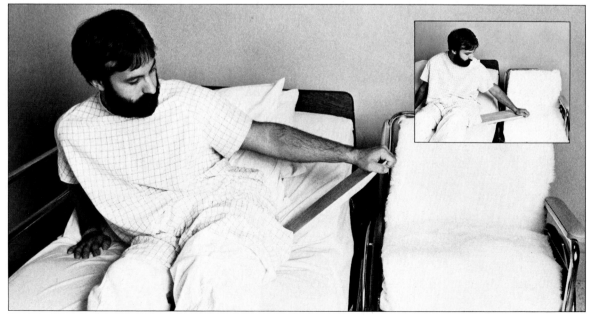

4 Next, he'll lift his buttocks and begin to inch his way across the board toward the wheelchair, as shown here. Tell Mr. Stafford to grasp the chair's left armrest with his left hand (see inset).

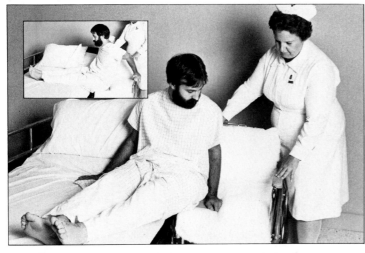

6 Now, have Mr. Stafford place his right hand on the transfer board, as shown in this photo. As he grasps the transfer board with his right hand, tell him to shift his weight to his left buttock.

Then instruct him to pull the board from underneath himself.

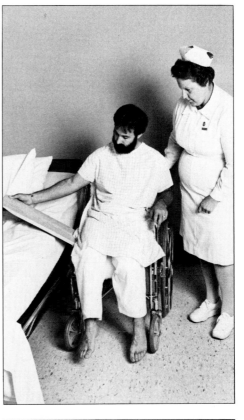

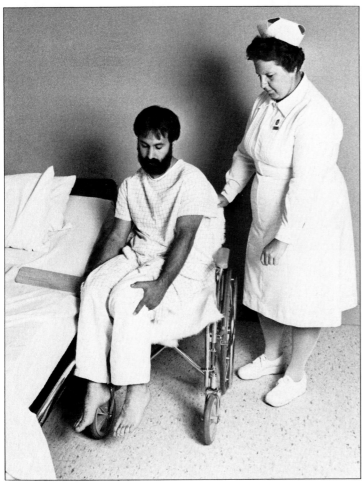

5 When Mr. Stafford reaches the chair, instruct him to guide his legs over the board and onto the chair.

7 Have Mr. Stafford put the armrests and legrests back onto the wheelchair.

Then, tell him to put on his socks and shoes.

Document your patient's instruction, progress, and tolerance, in your notes.

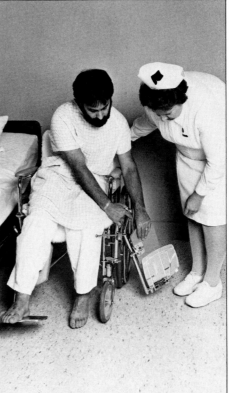

Positioning and exercise

Using the stand-pivot technique to transfer a patient from bed to wheelchair

1 *Consider this situation: Frank Shepard, a 56-year-old carpenter, has left-sided hemiplegia as the result of a cerebrovascular accident (CVA). When you check his chart, you see that the physical therapist has been teaching Mr. Shepard the stand-pivot transfer. Now you want to show Mrs. Shepard how to help her husband perform this transfer. Do you know how to proceed? Follow these steps:*

Begin reviewing the procedure with Mr. and Mrs. Shepard. Emphasize that this transfer can be performed easily at home. Have Mrs. Shepard watch as you help her husband perform the transfer. Then, lower the left side rail.

Now you're ready to position the left side of the wheelchair next to the left side of the bed.

· *Note:* Always position the wheelchair on the patient's unaffected side, if possible.

[Inset] Lock the wheels on the chair and the bed. If possible, detach the chair's legrests. Or, move them out of the way.

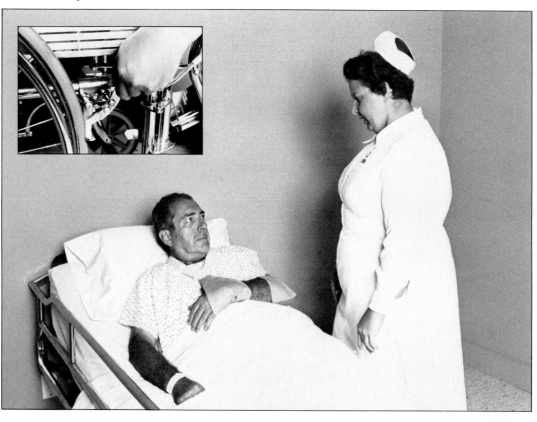

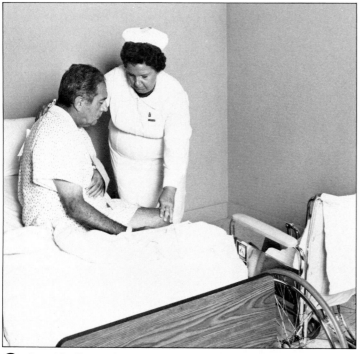

2 Seat Mr. Shepard on the edge of the bed, with his legs hanging over the side. Allow him time to regain his equilibrium. Put shoes on his feet and be sure his feet are touching the floor. If they aren't, lower the bed.

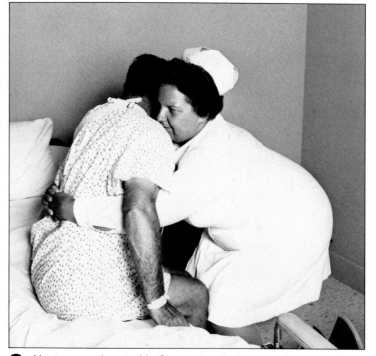

3 Next, move close to Mr. Shepard and place your knees against his knees, as the nurse is doing in this photo. Squat slightly and slide your arms under his arms. Then, lock your arms around his waist.

4 Instruct Mr. Shepard to lock his unaffected arm around your back.

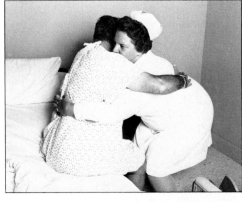

5 Ask Mr. Shepard to help you as much as possible. Push your knees against his to keep them stable. Then, assist him in reaching a standing position. Again, allow him a few seconds to regain his equilibrium.

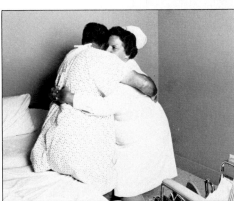

6 Now, pivot toward the wheelchair, as shown in this photo. Continue to support Mr. Shepard's knees with your knees as you turn his back toward the chair. Stop turning when your patient's back is directly in front of the wheelchair.

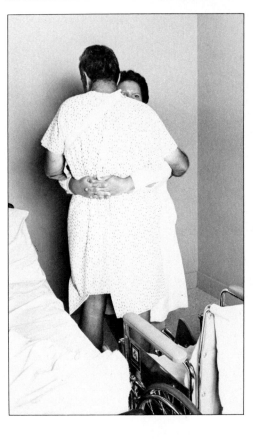

7 Instruct him to grasp the wheelchair's right armrest with his right hand.

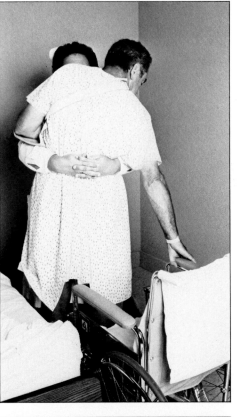

8 Then, as you squat down to lower him into the chair, he'll be able to guide himself into the seat.

Now, explain to Mrs. Shepard how she can arrange to rent or borrow a properly-equipped wheelchair for home use. Remember to tell her that the hospital's social service department may be able to help her obtain this equipment, but tell her that they may require a doctor's order.

Finally, document the procedure and any patient teaching in your nurses' notes.

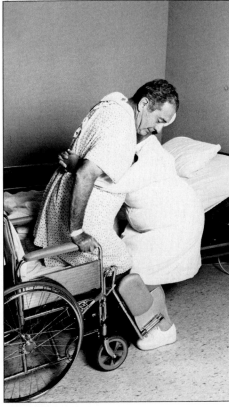

Positioning and exercise

Teaching your patient how to walk with a cane

1 *Let's imagine 65-year-old Martha Samuels has been transferred to your unit. She's experiencing left-sided weakness and unsteadiness from Parkinson's disease. Because Mrs. Samuels lives alone, the doctor instructs you to help Mrs. Samuels with her cane-walking. Here's what to do:*

Note: The patient in this photostory is using a Guardian Quadripoise® cane.

First, explain the procedure to Mrs. Samuels, and reassure her. Make sure she's wearing shoes and check that her cane is the right height.

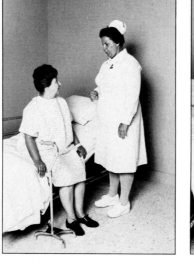

2 Have your patient slide to the edge of the bed and place her feet flat on the floor 6" (15.2 cm) apart. Help her into a standing position. Then, stand slightly to Mrs. Samuels' weakened side.

Now, instruct Mrs. Samuels to hold the cane in her right hand, with the tip about 4" (10.2 cm) to the side of her right foot. Tell her to distribute her weight evenly between her feet and the cane. Also remind her to keep the cane's rubber tips on the floor at all times.

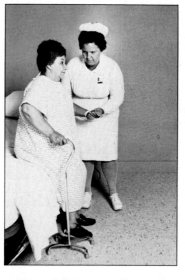

3 Instruct Mrs. Samuels to look ahead when she walks instead of looking at her feet. Then, ask your patient to shift her weight to her right leg as she moves the cane forward about 4" (10.2 cm).

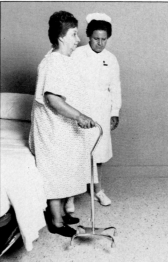

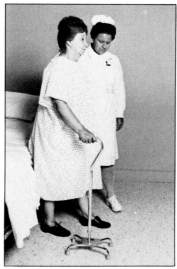

4 Next, with her weight supported on her right leg and the cane, have Mrs. Samuels move her left foot forward parallel with the cane, as shown here.

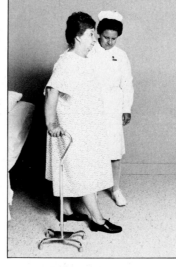

5 Tell Mrs. Samuels to shift her weight to her left leg and the cane, then move her right leg forward ahead of the cane, as shown. If she does this correctly, her heel will be slightly beyond the tip of the cane.

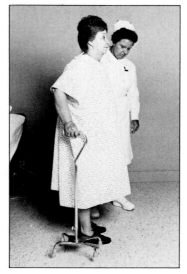

6 Now, tell Mrs. Samuels to move her left foot forward so it's even with her right foot, as shown here. Then instruct her to move her cane forward as instructed in step 3. Guide her through the above procedure several more times until you both feel she's ready to try it alone.

When Mrs. Samuels' family comes to visit, acquaint them with the proper procedure for cane-walking.

Document all patient teaching, along with your patient's progress in your nurses' notes.

Applying antiembolism stockings

1 *Are you caring for a neurologic patient who is confined to bed? If so, the doctor may order antiembolism stockings for your patient. As you know, these stockings compress superficial veins, minimizing the risk of thrombus formation. Do you know how to measure and apply the stockings properly? If you're unsure, follow these guidelines:*

First, have your patient lay flat in bed if she can tolerate it. Then, measure the largest part of her calf, as shown.

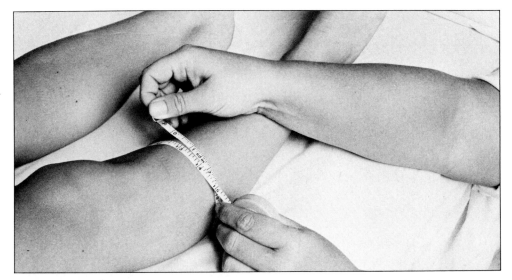

2 To fit knee-length stockings, measure from the back of your patient's knee to the bottom of her heel. For correct sizing, match these measurements with those on the manufacturer's card.

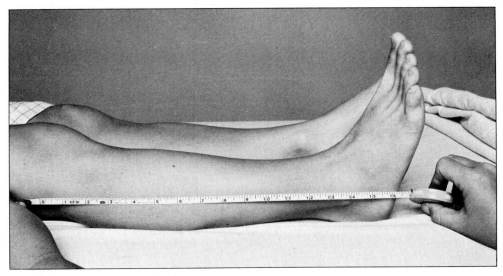

3 Has the doctor ordered waist-length stockings? If so, measure from her gluteal furrow down to her ankle. Also measure the largest part of her thigh (see inset).

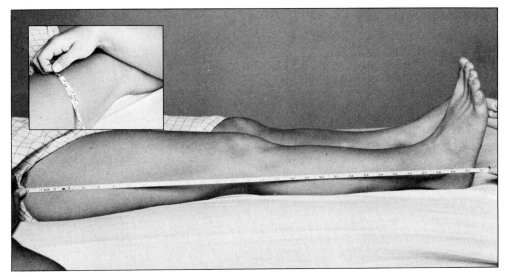

Positioning and exercise

Applying antiembolism stockings

4 Before you apply the stockings, check the circulation in your patient's legs. To do this, note color, appearance, and temperature. If they appear cool or cyanotic, notify the doctor before proceeding.

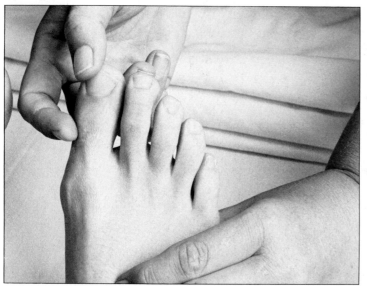

5 To apply the stockings, gather the stocking between your fingers from the top to the toes. Then, pull the stocking over the patient's toes, as shown here. Carefully pull the stocking up over the patient's ankle.

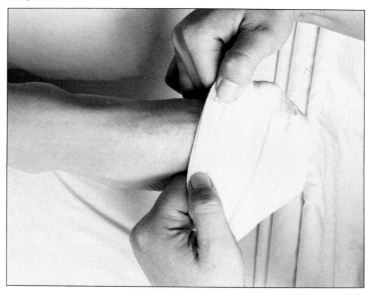

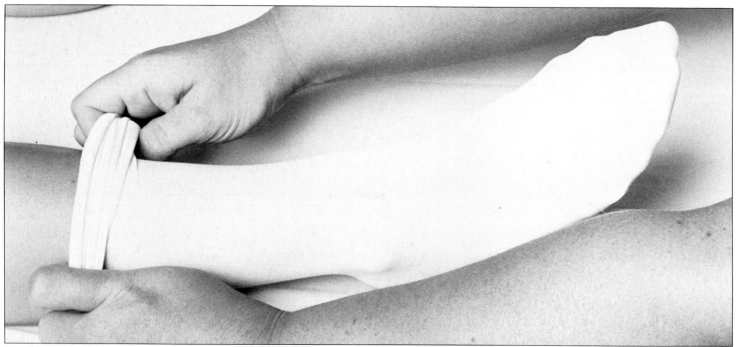

6 Now, unroll the remainder of the stocking over the patient's leg, as shown. Apply the other stocking following the same procedure. Be sure the stockings fit smoothly on the patient's legs. Wrinkles in the stockings may cause excessive pressure.

Are you applying waist-length stockings? If so, make sure you fit your patient with an adjustable belt. Check to be sure the belt's waistband or side panels don't press against a catheter, drainage tube, or incision. Then, attach the stockings to the belt.

Note: When both stockings are applied properly, elevate both legs so that they are above heart level to prevent stasis and clotting. If the stockings you've applied have toe holes, you'll be able to assess your patient's circulation more frequently.

Remove the stockings at least once every 24 hours. Doing so allows for circulatory and skin assessment, as well as allowing the legs to be washed. Check color, sensation, circulation, and ability to move. Notify the doctor if the patient complains of leg pain, has dusky-colored toenail beds, decreased or absent pedal pulses, or reddened areas. Document your findings in your nurses' notes.

Respiratory function

Nurses' guide to respiratory complications

If you've ever cared for a patient with a spinal cord injury, you know that respiratory therapy is very important. In fact, atelectasis and pneumonia are the most common complications of this neurologic disorder.

However, if you've ever performed respiratory therapy, you know there's more involved than suctioning a patient. The following pages will answer your questions about:
• suctioning when an artificial airway is in place.
• using an incentive spirometer.
• using intermittent positive pressure breathing (IPPB) therapy.
• complications that require special procedures.

But remember, respiratory therapy is so individualized we can only cover the basics here. For details on all the topics that follow, see the NURSING PHOTOBOOK PROVIDING RESPIRATORY CARE.

How familiar are you with respiratory complications associated with neurologic disorders? These complications may result from improper positioning, secretion aspiration associated with immobility, presence of a mucous plug or inadequate alveolar expansion. Do you know what signs and symptoms to look for and how to care for your patient properly? The following chart acquaints you with four common respiratory complications.

Follow these patient care guidelines:
• Turn and position your patient regularly, unless he's able to do so.
• Encourage your patient to deep breathe, fully expanding his lungs, and to cough.
• Observe and assess your patient's breath sounds and respiratory patterns, routinely.
• Administer intermittent positive pressure breathing (IPPB) treatments and incentive spirometry, if ordered.
• Percuss and vibrate your patient's chest to loosen secretions, as indicated.
• Explain all procedures to your patient.
• Provide emotional support for the patient and his family.

Complication	Signs and symptoms	Nursing intervention
Atelectasis (Incomplete expansion of alveoli or lung segments which may result in partial or total lung collapse)	• Sudden onset of dyspnea and cyanosis • Anxiety, apprehension • Elevated temperature • Tachycardia • Decreased chest expansion • Flatness on percussion • Sternal retractions • Diminished or absent breath sounds on auscultation • Drop in blood pressure • May be asymptomatic when developing slowly	• Encourage deep breathing exercises with inspiratory hold. • Position patient with the affected area in dependent position. • Administer antibiotics as ordered. • Encourage patient to drink plenty of fluids to loosen secretions. • Provide suctioning, as needed. • Be prepared to use mechanical ventilation. • Be ready to assist with bronchoscopy, if symptoms are not relieved by coughing or suctioning.
Pneumonia (Lung inflammation with consolidation; may result from aspiration)	• Dyspnea • Cough with production of thick, green, yellow, or rust sputum • Chest pain, especially in lateral lung fields; increased pain on inspiration • Shaking, chills • Fever, headache • Flushed skin • Chest dullness on palpation • Decreased breath sounds • Rales or rhonchi • Tachypnea	• Obtain sputum for culture and sensitivity, initially and periodically. • Administer antibiotics as ordered. • Provide complete bed rest. • Encourage patient to drink plenty of fluids to loosen secretions. • Perform tracheobronchial suctioning, following strict aseptic technique, as indicated.
Pulmonary edema (Extravascular fluid accumulation in pulmonary tissues and air spaces which may result from a lesion of the hypothalamus or medulla)	• Severe dyspnea, and paroxysmal nocturnal dyspnea • Rales, wheezing • Cold, clammy skin • Thready pulse • Tachycardia and tachypnea • Altered consciousness level, may range from confusion to agitation • Decreased blood pressure • Cough with production of sputum which may be blood-tinged	• Administer oxygen at high rate, unless contraindicated. • Monitor patient carefully. Check central venous pressure (CVP) line and cardiac leads frequently. If patient's receiving IPPB therapy, look for signs of increased intracranial pressure. Remember, IPPB therapy may aggravate intracranial vascular congestion. • Place patient in high Fowler's position and provide complete bed rest. • Monitor patient's intake and output closely. • Administer diuretics, as ordered. • Provide patient with a sodium-restricted diet, as ordered. • Administer cardiac drugs as ordered. • Be ready to apply rotating tourniquets, as ordered. • Be prepared to assist with endotracheal tube insertion and mechanical ventilation, as needed. • Prepare patient for hemodialysis, if indicated.
Bronchospasm (Spasmodic contraction of bronchi muscle resulting from suctioning of an allergic reaction, causing mucous edema and increased mucus secretions)	• Coughing, wheezing, dyspnea • Intermittent low-grade fever, especially at night • Tenacious and purulent sputum with brown flecks or plugs	• Administer bronchodilator, steroids, and antibiotics, as ordered. • Monitor arterial blood gas measurements. • Provide bed rest.

Learning about incentive spirometers

A patient with neuromuscular weakness, or any other type of neurologic disorder, is especially susceptible to pooling of secretions, and alveolar collapse. To help minimize these respiratory complications, the doctor may order an incentive spirometer for your patient.

As you may know, an incentive spirometer helps mobilize secretions, and promotes expectoration by coughing. But keep in mind that the spirometer also maintains inhalation volumes, allowing for alveolar inflation.

How does an incentive spirometer work? The air a patient inhales through the flowtube is measured by the lights on the spirometer panel. When the patient inhales sufficient air to achieve the goal set by his doctor or inhalation therapist, a light on the panel blinks. As the patient holds his breath, the blinking light stays lit and the HOLD light comes on. The HOLD light stays on for 2.5 seconds after the patient stops inhaling. However, if he's able to continue inhalation, the light will go past the goal reached, establishing a new goal for the patient.

The Spirocare® Incentive Breathing Exerciser, shown here, measures up to 5,500 ml of air flow. It has three volume range settings with an adjustable scale from one to ten within each range. This model also features disposable flowtubes to minimize the risk of cross-contamination.

Now, read the photostory that follows to learn how to operate this incentive spirometer.

How to use an incentive spirometer

1 *Are you showing your patient how to use a Spirocare® Incentive Breathing Exerciser? If so, here's how to proceed:* First, explain the procedure to your patient. Then, press the POWER switch to ON. Now, slide the VOLUME RANGE switch at the back of the unit to the LOW setting. By doing this, the unit will measure approximately 250 to 1,375 ml of air flow (increased at 125 ml volume increments) as ordered by the patient's doctor.

Low	250 to 1,375 ml
Medium	500 to 2,750 ml
High	1,000 to 5,500 ml

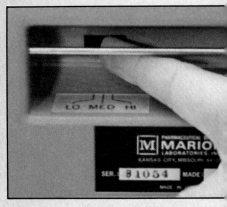

2 Suppose your patient's doctor has ordered an inhalation goal of 750 ml of air flow. To set this goal, rotate the black dial at the right of the cord attachment toward you until a blinking red light appears at 5 on the volume scale. Remember, when your patient inhales, this goal will be indicated by the blinking light.

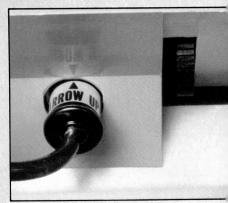

3 Firmly hold the flowtube's short, flanged end in your right hand. Next, pull downward on the plastic with your left hand, as you push the flowtube upward with your right hand. Continue to unwrap the flowtube's long barrel. But remember, to prevent the possibility of contamination, keep the short, flanged end wrapped.

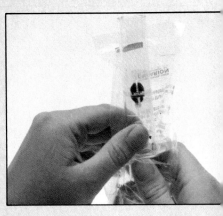

4 Now, grasping the flowtube holder with your left hand, insert the flowtube's long end into the holder. Rotate the short, flanged end until the nipple catches in the holder slot, as shown here. Make sure the flowtube fits firmly in the holder.

Being careful not to touch the flanged end, remove the remaining plastic.

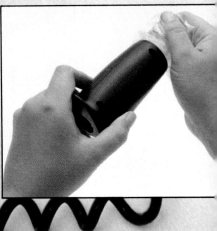

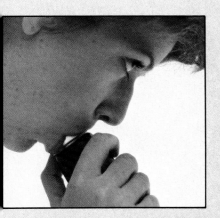

5 Instruct your patient to wrap her fingers firmly around the flowtube holder. Her thumb should overlap the edge of the clear plastic flange. Check to be sure the mouthpiece is clear and unobstructed. Press the GOALS ACHIEVED RESET button before proceeding. Now, have your patient exhale normally. Then, tell her to place her mouth tightly around the flowtube up to the flange (see photo).

6 Tell your patient that the blinking red light at 6 identifies her inhalation goal. Explain that when she inhales, another red light will appear opposite the number 1 and begin climbing the scale. If she reaches her goal, the red light will climb to 6, and the blinking light at 6 will become momentarily constant. If your patient surpasses her goal, the constant red light will climb past the blinking light.

Instruct your patient to inhale deeply enough to force the number 6 light to blink. Now, encourage her to hold her breath for several seconds until the blinking light becomes constant and the HOLD light shines yellow. When the HOLD light goes out, have your patient remove the flowtube from her mouth and exhale normally. Remember to praise her for her effort.

Repeat this exercise five times, as ordered by the doctor. Remind your patient to rest between each exercise.

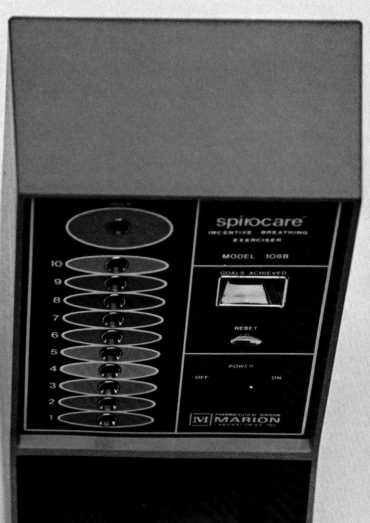

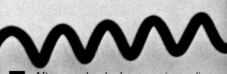

7 After each day's exercise, dispose of the flowtube, following infection control standards. Then, rotate the black dial at the right of the cord attachment to 0. Press the RESET button, and turn the POWER switch to OFF.

Finally, document the date, time, and patient's inhalation volume, as well as her tolerance to the exercise, in your notes.

Respiratory function

Percussing a patient's lungs

1 *Fifty-year-old Claude Maxwell was admitted to your unit with myasthenia gravis. Now, Mr. Maxwell has developed pneumonia in the middle and lower lobes of his lungs. The doctor's ordered chest percussion performed every 4 hours. As you know, chest percussion dislodges thick, tenacious secretions from your patient's bronchial walls so that they can be expectorated or suctioned. Do you know how to perform chest percussion properly? These photos will show you.*

Caution: In certain neurologic patients, such as a patient with increased intracranial pressure (ICP), chest percussion may be contraindicated.

First, explain to Mr. Maxwell what you're going to do. Then, elevate the foot of the bed 15°.

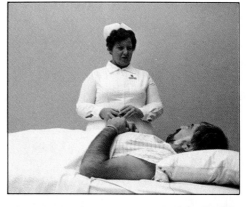
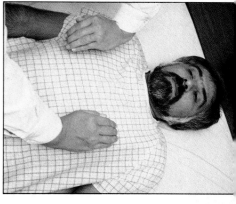

2 Now, you're ready to drain the superior and inferior segments of the lingula of the left lung. Position your patient so he's lying partly on his back and partly on his right side. Tuck a pillow

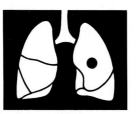

under his left side for support. Then, locate the fourth and sixth ribs on the left side of his chest by feeling just above and below the nipple line. Beginning between the fourth and sixth ribs, percuss for 3 to 5 minutes before changing your patient's position.

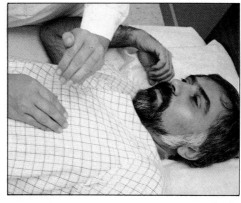
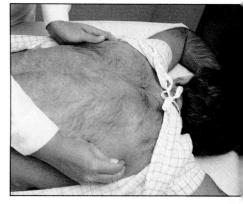

3 Now, position your patient so he's lying partly on his back and partly on his left side, as shown here. Tuck a pillow under his back for support. Next, percuss the right side of his chest be-

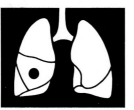

tween the fourth and sixth ribs. Doing so will help drain the right lung's middle lobe.

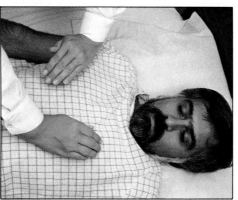
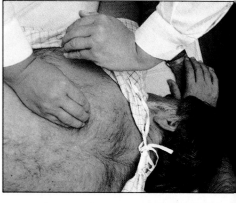

4 To drain the superior segments of both lower lobes, place the bed in a flat position. Place your patient on his abdomen. Then, as shown here, percuss both sides of his back over the lower ends of his scapulae.

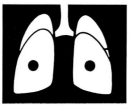
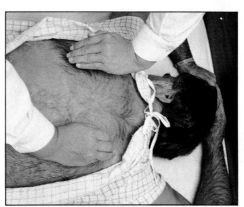
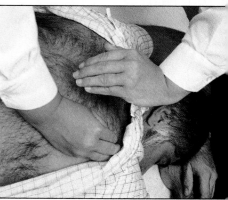

5 To drain the anterior basal segments of both lower lobes, elevate the foot of the bed 30°. Position Mr. Maxwell on his back, and percuss both sides of his chest. But remember, do not percuss the center of his chest, over his stomach, as it may cause pain and damage.

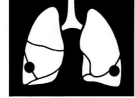

Important: An acutely ill patient may have trouble breathing in this position. Adjust the bed angle to one the patient can tolerate, before beginning percussion.

6 Keeping the foot of the bed elevated 30°, position your patient on his abdomen. Percuss both sides of his back at the tenth rib level and above, as shown here. Be careful not to percuss over his kidneys, located below the tenth rib level, as this may cause pain and damage.

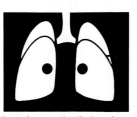

7 Now, to drain the lateral basal segment of the left lower lobe, position your patient so he's lying partly on his abdomen and partly on his right side, as shown here. Then, percuss his left side at the tenth rib level and above.

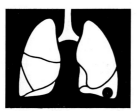

8 To drain the lateral basal segment of the right lower lobe, position Mr. Maxwell so that he is lying partly on his abdomen and partly on his left side. Then, percuss his right side, as the nurse is doing here, at the tenth rib level and above.

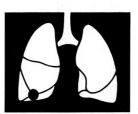

Document the entire procedure in your nurses' notes.

Understanding IPPB therapy

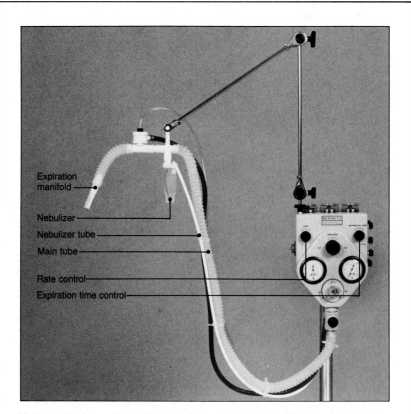

Expiration manifold

Nebulizer

Nebulizer tube

Main tube

Rate control

Expiration time control

You're caring for a patient with a spinal cord lesion. Because of severe pain, the patient's unable to deep breathe. To help minimize respiratory complications, the doctor orders intermittent positive pressure breathing (IPPB) therapy.

Keep in mind that IPPB therapy helps promote bronchodilation, loosen secretions, reduce pulmonary edema, and can deliver deep aerosol therapy. Here's how it works:

A ventilator, set at a prescribed pressure, forces humidified air or nebulized medication through the tubing. Your patient inhales the air or medication through a mouthpiece attached to the tubing. As he inhales, the positive pressure inflates his lungs.

Caution: Never give your patient a dry IPPB treatment. Use sterile distilled water or normal saline solution to provide humidity if a specific medication is not ordered by the doctor.

When he's inhaled sufficient air or medication, and the preset pressure is reached, the ventilator shuts off, and your patient removes his mouthpiece. Then, tell him to exhale completely. As he exhales, he'll release the positive pressure, helping mobilize secretions. Have your patient repeat this proce-

dure for 10 to 15 minutes, or as tolerated, each session.

Be sure to remind your patient that he may experience episodes of coughing following IPPB therapy. Assure him the coughing is normal and beneficial.

Remember: To ensure effective IPPB treatment, the patient's lips should form a tight seal around the mouthpiece.

In addition, you'll need to closely monitor your patient during and after IPPB therapy for the following signs and symptoms:
* nausea
* tremors or dizziness
* rapid, shallow respirations
* distended abdomen
* sudden drop in blood pressure accompanied by increasing heart rate.

If you see any of these signs, discontinue the treatment and notify the doctor. He may want to stop IPPB therapy. Also, familiarize yourself with the drug you're administering by IPPB therapy. Observe the patient closely for any adverse effects produced by the specific drug.

Document the procedure, all observations, time, and the patient's tolerance to the treatment, in your nurses' notes.

Respiratory function

How to use a vaporizer: some tips

Your patient wih a tracheostomy is being discharged, and the doctor has ordered a vaporizer to be placed in his room at home. Why? Because moisturized air produced by the vaporizer loosens thick secretions that may pool in your patient's respiratory system.

You'll want to review the procedure for setting up and caring for a vaporizer with the patient and his family. Tell them to follow these guidelines:
• Place the vaporizer on a table several feet from the bed. Be sure the steam's directed toward your patient.
• Gather the prescribed medication and a container of distilled water.
• Fill the vaporizer with the distilled water to the level marked on the unit. Then, plug in the vaporizer.
• Measure the correct dosage of medication, then pour it into the water or vaporizer cup.
• Keep several feet between the vaporizer and the patient to ensure his comfort and to avoid accidental burns. Instruct the family to periodically check the patient while the vaporizer's on.
• Replace any damp linen, as needed.
• Continue to use the vaporizer as indicated or prescribed.

Preparing your patient to receive oxygen therapy at home

The doctor wants your patient, who has suffered hypoxia following a severe head injury, to continue receiving oxygen therapy at home.

Although many suppliers provide instructions on how to operate oxygen therapy equipment, you'll want to review oxygen therapy guidelines with the patient and his family. Demonstrate the following: how to connect a flowmeter and regulator; how to properly connect an oxygen cylinder; and how to set up a humidifier.

Make sure your patient and his family understand what you've told them. Keep your directions simple. Ask the family to repeat each demonstration after you've finished to clear up any confusion they might have. Remember to document what you've done in the patient's discharge summary and your nurses' notes.

To help your patient and his family remember all your instructions at home, give them a copy of the home care aid below.

Home care

How to care for oxygen

Dear Patient:
To help you breathe more easily, your doctor wants you to continue using oxygen at home. Follow these instructions when using oxygen at home.
• Rent or buy the oxygen therapy equipment you'll need. If you're able to move around, and need oxygen all the time, you'll want to obtain a portable unit in addition to your main source.
• Always keep at least a 3-day supply of oxygen on hand. Plan ahead and prepare for any long holiday weekends when your supplier will be closed. If you decide on oxygen with a continuous electrical source, talk to your supplier about getting a small emergency tank to use in case of a power failure.
• Be sure your supplier teaches you and your family how to change oxygen cylinders properly.
• Make sure a NO SMOKING sign's posted on the door of the house and of the room you're occupying.
• Make your family and visitors aware of oxygen's hazards and the precautions they should take.
• Use your common sense when using electrical appliances, such as radios and television. Check to be sure all appliances are properly grounded and the wires are in good condition.

• To prevent the possibility of electrical shock or sparks, avoid close contact with electrical appliances.
• Keep all oxygen containers away from electrical baseboard vents, gas or kerosene heaters, radiators, stoves, and grills.
• Close all valves when the oxygen's not in use, even on an oxygen container that registers empty.
• Adjust the cylinder's flowmeter so you're receiving _____ liters of oxygen per minute.
• Add water to the humidifier as necessary to maintain the proper water level. However, change all water in the container daily.
• Clean the ends of your nasal cannula daily. Use water-soluble ointments to lubricate your nostrils. Never use oil-based products, such as mineral oil, or flammable products, such as rubbing alcohol.
• Advise a family member to call your doctor immediately if you develop any of the following signs and symptoms: increased trouble breathing; irregular breathing; rapid heartbeat; blue lips or nailbeds; confusion; or restlessness.
• If the family member's unable to reach your doctor, have him take you to the nearest emergency room.

Bowel and bladder function

Loss of bowel and bladder control is one of the most devastating problems for a patient with brain or spinal cord damage. Helping a patient attain continency is one of the challenges of neurologic nursing.

How familiar are you with the various methods available to help a patient gain continence? For example, do you know how to plan a bladder management program? Or how a timed-voiding program works? Do you know how to initiate reflex stimulation techniques? Can you perform Credé's maneuver?

Do you know the importance of providing a proper diet for a patient with a bowel or bladder problem? Or how to stimulate the bowel?

In this section, we'll answer these questions and provide additional information that'll help you properly care for a patient with a bowel or bladder dysfunction.

Learning about bladder and bowel programs

Teaching your patient with a neurologic disorder proper bladder and bowel training will help him attain his full potential. As you know, you'll want to begin planning a bladder and bowel management program as soon as possible.

First, explain to your patient how his disorder affects continence. Review normal bladder and bowel functioning with him, then explain how his neurologic disorder alters the reflexes and senses that control his urine and stool evacuation.

As you talk to your patient, assess his physical, social, and emotional concerns regarding incontinence. How, for example, is his disorder affecting his bladder and bowel functioning? What were his previous bladder and bowel habits? How much has the dysfunctioning affected his lifestyle? Does the incontinence embarrass him?

Then, prepare a management program based on your patient's needs and concerns. When you do, consider his mobility, motivation, and economic resources. Also, evaluate his family's desire to cooperate. After you've prepared the program, familiarize your patient and his family with the various methods that may help him attain regularity and continence. Discuss with your patient the methods he's most comfortable performing. Then, before he leaves the hospital, be sure to instruct your patient and family in all parts of his program; for example, the Valsalva maneuver and Credé's maneuver, and reflex bladder and bowel stimulation techniques.

As you provide day-to-day nursing care, remember to ensure your patient's privacy during his daily bladder and bowel routines. In addition, maintain communication with your patient and his family as you reevaluate his management program's effectiveness. Revise his program, as necessary.

Understanding bladder management

As you know, the normal bladder acts as a storage vessel, expanding as it fills with urine. This distention stimulates stretch receptors in the bladder wall, sending impulses to the spinal cord's sacral portion. These impulses initiate the micturition reflex, forcing bladder contraction and dilation of the urethral sphincters. Impulses from the micturition reflex also reach the cerebral cortex.

An efferent message from the brain can contract the external sphincter, stopping urination. However, brain or spinal cord damage disrupts communication with the bladder, causing dysfunction and incontinence.

Prepare a bladder management program as soon as possible for the incontinent patient, based on these objectives:
• preventing overdistention
• preserving normal bladder capacity and muscle tone
• establishing a routine pattern of elimination which requires minimum use of artificial devices or procedures (such as a catheter or stoma)
• prevention of infection
• allowing for the patient's ease and comfort in his environment.

Keep in mind that bladder management programs are aimed at balancing the forces of bladder expulsion and the forces of resistance. Urodynamics, a series of bladder tests, helps adequately diagnose bladder expulsion and resistive forces. This enables the doctor to correctly prescribe treatment based on physiologic principles. Then, bladder management can be established by combining your patient's goals with the results of the following urodynamic tests:
• *Electromyography (EMG)* evaluates striated external sphincter function while relaxed, and assesses contraction of the voluntary sphincter and detrusor urinae.
• *Urethral pressure profile* evaluates bladder neck and urethral smooth muscle functioning.
• *Cystometry* evaluates detrusor function based on sensation, pressure volume responses, reflex detrusor urinae contractions, and the voluntary ability to suppress detrusor contraction.
• *Uroflowmetry* evaluates urethral and bladder function by giving normal or abnormal flow rate readings.

After you've assessed the degree of your patient's bladder dysfunctioning through the urodynamic test results, you're ready to establish a management program. Use one of the following methods based on its success of bringing your patient toward proper bladder functioning:
• *Time voiding:* Toileting on a regular schedule; for example, as soon as he arises in the morning, after meals, and before any physical activities, such as occupational therapy. If your patient is incontinent between toiletings, adjust his schedule accordingly.

Note: An alternative method of timed voiding may be toileting every 2 hours.

In addition, encourage your patient to drink large amounts of fluids (about 2,500 ml every 24 hours). Provide most of his fluids before his final daily meal to alleviate urinating in large amounts during the night. When it's time for your patient to urinate, assist him to a commode chair or toilet. Avoid using a bedpan, which contributes to incomplete bladder emptying and may cause undue pressure over the ischial tuberosity and sacrum.

To help your patient initiate urination, use the following methods: running water, giving him a drink, and having him bear down.
• *External urinary collecting devices:* To meet your patient's needs, try to find the correct combination of latex sheath, fastener, and collection bag to ensure proper drainage without urine leakage.
• *External compression:* Abdominal strain, Valsalva and Credé's maneuver all increase intravesical pressure, promoting urinary flow.

Important: To ensure that your patient's urinary tract can safely handle external compression, be sure urodynamic testing's performed before proceeding with either of these methods.

If using abdominal strain, or the Valsalva maneuver, have your patient sit on a toilet or commode chair. Ask him to inhale deeply and hold his breath. Then, have him push down hard, as in bearing down for a bowel movement.

Bowel and bladder function

Understanding bladder management continued

• *Reflex stimulation techniques:* Sacral or lumbar dermatome stimulation in a patient with an upper motor lesion provokes a reflex contraction of the bladder. To stimulate reflex activity, you may do any one of the following: tapping his suprapubic area; stroking his glans penis, thighs, or vulva; anal dilatation; tugging his pubic hairs; and flexing his toes. To stimulate his suprapubic area, begin with taps of high intensity and long duration. And remember, as the training program continues, stimulus needed to produce urinating decreases in duration and intensity.

Caution: Avoid excessive force that may damage his skin.

Encourage your patient to learn self-stimulation of the bladder.

As you know, patients on an intermittent catheterization program should perform reflex stimulation between catheterization periods.

• *Intermittent catheterization program:* This allows for an unrestricted urine flow from the kidneys, keeps the catheter out of the bladder for a greater length of time, and prevents excessive urine collection in the bladder.

Caution: Intermittent catheterization is contraindicated in vesicoureteral reflex; hydronephrosis; acute or chronic pyelonephritis; severe cystitis; calculi in the urinary tract; and major structural changes in the urethra.

Restrict your patient's fluid intake to 1,800 to 2,000 ml from 8 a.m. to 8 p.m. Then, begin catheterizing your patient at 4 hour intervals. If the residual volume is greater than 400 ml, decrease catheterizations to every 3 hours. Continue assessing time intervals by the amount of residual urine in the bladder.

When the volume of urine is 100 to 150 ml, gradually increase the intervals between catheterizations. This process can take from 2 to 3 months, up to 1 year following the onset of a neurogenic bladder problem.

• *Continuous drainage:* Any external device draining urine from a patient's bladder, such as an indwelling (Foley) or condom catheter connected to a straight closed drainage system.

• *Surgical procedures:* May include suprapubic catheterization or an ostomy, such as an ileostomy or ileal conduit, to provide continuous urine drainage.

Performing Credé's maneuver

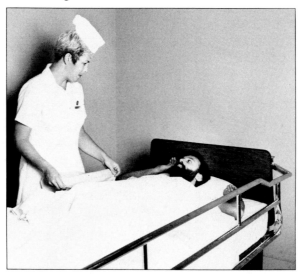

1 *Credé's maneuver is a commonly used external compression technique. Do you know how to perform this maneuver properly? If you're unsure, follow these steps:*

First, gather the equipment: a urinal for your male patient or a bedpan for your female patient, or an external urinary collecting device.

Place him in a supine position. Then, explain the procedure to your patient.

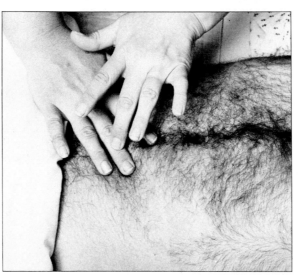

2 Next, begin palpating his bladder to determine location and height. Then, as you percuss his bladder, expect to hear dull sounds, indicating bladder fullness.

Note: Percussing an empty bladder produces a hollow sound.

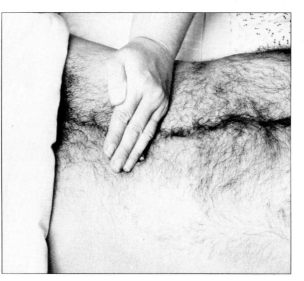

3 Now you're ready to begin Credé's maneuver. Place your fingers at the top of your patient's bladder, as the nurse is doing here.

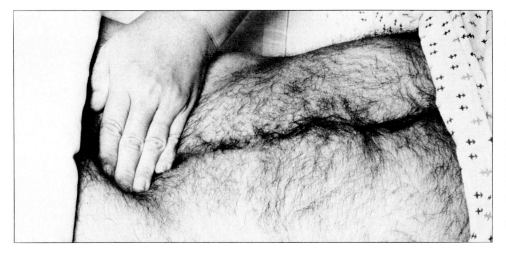

4 Slowly, knead your patient's bladder with your fingers, as shown, applying progressive pressure.

Caution: Avoid grinding your fingers on your patient's skin. Doing so may cause irritation or ulcerations.

If performed properly, Credé's maneuver initiates urination. Stop urination by removing your fingers from his abdomen. To determine the amount of urine remaining, palpate the bladder again. If urine's still present, reapply progressive pressure. Make sure you completely empty the bladder. Urine remaining in the bladder can lead to renal complications; for example, infection.

Document the procedure and the amount of urine obtained, in your notes.

Understanding suprapubic catheterization

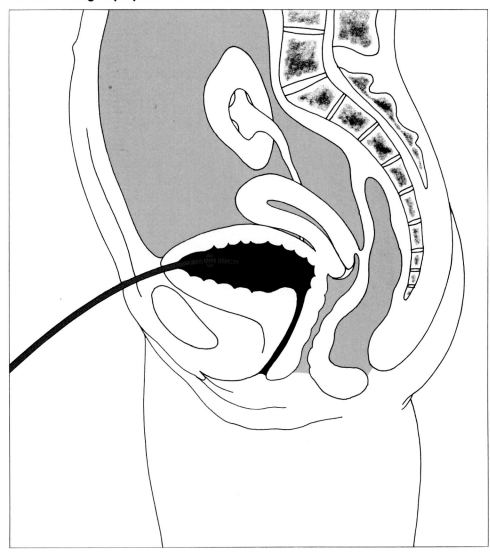

Let's say you're caring for a patient with a T_6 spinal transection which has compromised her ability to urinate. To provide urinary drainage, the doctor orders suprapubic catheterization.

Keep in mind that a suprapubic catheter allows you to easily evaluate your patient's ability to urinate, is less likely to cause urinary tract infections, and may be more comfortable for her than a urethral catheter. (For more information on urethral catheterization, see the NURSING PHOTOBOOK IMPLEMENTING UROLOGIC PROCEDURES.)

The doctor may perform suprapubic catheterization at your patient's bedside. What's your role? To prepare your patient for the procedure, assist the doctor during the procedure, and care for your patient and the catheter following the procedure.

Here's how to proceed: Begin by explaining the procedure and why it's necessary to your patient. Tell her that you'll prep her skin with povidone-iodine solution. Then the doctor will inject a local anesthetic into the suprapubic area.

To perform the insertion, the doctor will make a small surgical incision in the suprapubic area. Then, he'll insert a trocar and cannula into the bladder. When the trocar and cannula are in place, he'll remove the trocar, feed the catheter through the cannula, and then remove the cannula (see illustration).

Next, he'll attach the catheter to a closed drainage system. Then, he'll either suture the catheter in place or secure it with a commercially-made retention body seal.

Now, follow these care guidelines:
• Always wash your hands before and after touching the catheter and drainage bag.
• Check the catheter for proper drainage;

Bowel and bladder function

Understanding suprapubic catheterization continued

empty the the drainage bag every 8 hours, using aseptic techinque.
• Note the color, consistency, and amount of urine. If the urine appears bloody, your patient may have an internal injury or a bowel perforation caused during insertion. Notify the doctor immediately.
• To prevent urine flow blockage, check the drainage tubing to make sure it's not kinked, looped, or obstructed. As you know, an obstruction can be caused by improper positioning (the catheter tip pressed against the bladder wall); a blood clot; sediment; or tubing flaw. If you suspect an obstruction, notify the doctor. He'll either reposition the tube, try to clear it by irrigation, or replace it.
• Provide adequate fluid intake, as ordered, to prevent residual urine pooling and possible infection.
• Give the patient ascorbic acid, as ordered, to acidify her urine and inhibit microorganism growth.
• Secure the drainage bag at the side of the bed so it remains below your patient's bladder level. Always keep the bag off the floor to prevent contamination.
• Change the insertion site dressing daily, or more frequently if soiled or wet, following strict aseptic technique.
• Avoid clamping the tube. If you must clamp the tube; for example, to obtain a urine specimen, do so briefly.
• Irrigate your patient's catheter only as ordered. Irrigation irritates delicate tissue and may cause infection. Discard a disposable irrigation set after one use.

When your patient regains her ability to urinate, the doctor will order the catheter removed. Because the surgical incision is small, suturing after catheter removal is usually unnecessary. Following strict aseptic technique, cleanse the incision, and apply an adhesive bandage strip.

Suppose your patient fails to regain her ability to urinate. In this case, the doctor may order urinary diversion surgery to create an ostomy. An enterostomal therapist will prepare the patient. However, if your hospital doesn't have one on staff, you'll need to prepare your patient by explaining the surgery as well as proper stoma care and ostomy pouch management. (For more information, see the NURSING PHOTOBOOK PERFORMING GI PROCEDURES.)

Learning about bowel management

In normal bowel functioning, end products of food begin as fluids in the ascending colon, and solidify as the colon absorbs water and electrolytes, creating fecal matter and gas. Then, fecal matter mixes in the colon and is moved into the rectum. Gas and feces in the rectum cause distention, initiating the defecation reflex. This reflex relaxes the internal sphincter, and tightens the external sphincter. Remember, the internal sphincter responds involuntarily to a reflex action caused by distention.

Now, a message is sent to the brain to defecate, causing the external sphincter to relax and the anal sphincter to contract. This permits the sigmoid colon and rectum to empty. However, defecation can be prohibited by voluntarily constricting the external sphincter.

In patients with some neurologic disorders, voluntary sphincter control is impaired, blocking normal defecation. This impairment causes incontinence and constipation.

Establishing a bowel routine is an important part of managing bowel dysfunction. A bowel management program should have two objectives: regularity and continence. Plan a program that incorporates all of the following:
• Proper diet: Provide your patient with a diet high in fluid and roughage, such as lettuce and bran. Discourage eating refined foods, such as pastries and white bread, which can cause constipation.
• Bowel medications: Use stool softeners, laxatives which stimulate the bowel, and bulk formers. You may also need to give your patient a suppository, which promotes peristalsis and smooth stool passage.
• Physical activity: Gravity and change of body position can help move the stool out of the body. Activity increases peristalsis through muscle tone. Turn your patient frequently if he can't change his body position. Unless contraindicated, get him to sit in a chair, or stand with assistance. Abdominal exercises or splinting can increase intra-abdominal pressure, causing the stool to descend past the anal sphincter.
• Timed procedures: For defecation, choose a time that's convenient for your patient, and then try to maintain this time each day that the bowel routine's performed.

If your patient's had a cerebrovascular accident (CVA), schedule his bowel routine when his gastrocolic reflex is most active; for example, ½ hour after a meal. For a patient with a spinal cord injury, a morning routine before his occupational therapy class might be a good choice.

Performing bowel stimulation

You can establish a bowel program through digital stimulation of the rectum. Here's how to perform this procedure.

Begin by obtaining a doctor's order to initiate the procedure, if necessary. Set up and maintain a regular time to perform the stimulation. Then, assemble the equipment you'll need: two or three bed-saver pads; a paper bag; water-soluble lubricant; soap; basin; washcloth and towel; and a glove. Before positioning your patient, place the bed-saver pads on the bed and wash your hands.

Now, place your patient in either a left Sims' position (lying on his left side with his left leg extended and right knee and thigh drawn up), or place him on a bowel stimulation chair.

About 30 to 40 minutes before bowel stimulation, you'll need to insert a suppository.

Note: If your patient has a fecal impaction, remove the impaction before inserting the suppository.

Then, put on your glove and lubricate your gloved finger. Insert your gloved finger ½" to 1" (1.3 to 2.5 cm) into the patient's rectum. After you move your finger in a rotating motion, gently pull the rectum to one side. Allow 15 minutes for the stool to empty. If any bleeding occurs, stop immediately and notify the doctor. If, after 15 minutes, his stool hasn't emptied, wait 24 hours before repeating the procedure.

After completing the procedure, remove and dispose of your glove, following your hospital's policy. Then, cleanse the patient's perineal area with soap and water, and dry it thoroughly. Remove the soiled bed-saver pads and dispose of them in the paper bag, following your hospital's policy. Wash your hands.

Document the color, consistency, and amount of stool obtained.

Note: Several days after establishing your patient's daily bowel program, you may find that his stool resists moving when the procedure's performed. In this situation, try performing the bowel program on alternate days, or every third day.

Sexual function

Sexual apprehensions may be one of your patient's fears after learning of his neurologic disorder. Unless you're able to quickly recognize and deal with your patient's sexual anxiety, he may lose all interest in himself, his family, and his rehabilitation.

In the next two pages, we'll discuss various methods of helping your patient cope with his sexuality and sexual function. We'll familiarize you with some alternate sexual positions and mechanical aids. You'll also find some valuable information you can pass on to your patient. Study this information carefully.

Helping your patient cope with sexuality and sexual function

In time, a patient with a neurologic disorder may develop sexual apprehensions. Because his feelings of sexuality are so closely tied to self-image and self-worth, anything that alters that image may damage his sense of fulfillment.

Prior to his neurologic disorder, your patient may not have thought much about his sexuality and sexual function. Now he may feel the need to assess his feelings about his own sexuality and discuss them with someone.

As a nurse, you probably spend more time with your patient during this period of adjustment than any other person. As you develop a rapport with your patient, encourage him to express his feelings.

But first, you'll need to establish and deal with your own feelings about sex. Of course, you have your own perceptions of sexuality based on your environmental, cultural, educational, and religious background. But, regardless of your feelings, you'll need to remain open-minded when dealing with a patient whose values, sexual practices, and preferences may differ from your own.

Learn as much as possible about your patient's neurologic disorder, as well as how it may affect him sexually. Be prepared to explain how his nervous system has been damaged, and what level of sexual function he can expect. Use terms he can understand.

If you feel uncomfortable discussing sexuality and sexual function with your patient, ask a co-worker or family member who feels comfortable dealing with the subject to take over for you. Remember, any feelings of embarrassment, disapproval, or inadequacy you have will be projected to your patient.

Keep in mind that your patient's reaction to sex depends on his environmental, cultural, educational, and religious background. He may view himself as being of little value to anyone. He may have

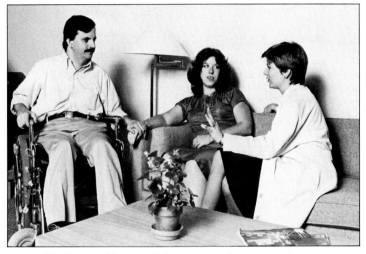

fears of being unable to satisfy his partner. He may also deny that sexuality is part of his life, or he may feel that a part of his life is gone forever.

Your patient may be apprehensive or anxious about sharing sexual information with you. Introduce the topic of sexuality in a private, nonthreatening manner. Make your questions open-ended, such as:
• Do you see yourself as having changed because of your disorder? In what ways?
• What will be different in your life because of your disorder?
• How do you feel your disorder will affect your sexual function?
• Did you have a sexual relationship before your disorder?
• Who are the important people in your life? What type of relationship do you have with these people?

As you talk to your patient, note his verbal, as well as his nonverbal, reactions. Remember, facial expressions may tell you a lot about what your patient's feeling.

Try to anticipate your patient's questions and be prepared to answer them truthfully and calmly. If your patient confronts you with a question you can't answer because you're uncomfortable or unfamiliar with the subject matter, tell him you'll get the information for him. And be sure to obtain the information as soon as possible. Here are some questions your patient

may ask:
• How can I have sex when I can't move?
• Why have sex if I can't feel anything?
• Can I have an erection?
• Who would want to have a sexual relationship with me?

Allow your patient some time to talk about his feelings and concerns. But never answer questions about sexuality for him. Encourage him to discuss his fears and concerns with his sexual partner.

Remember, both patient and partner will face difficult adjustments and may benefit from professional sexual counseling. If necessary, refer them to experts in the field.

Encourage your patient and his partner to experiment with various sexual methods and techniques. Tell them they'll probably attain a satisfactory sex life in time. But remind them that whatever sexual activity they engage in must be comfortable physically and emotionally for both parties. They must feel that sex—whatever form it takes for them— is normal: an expression of themselves, and of their desire to share intimacy.

Above all, encourage your patient to be open and honest with his sexual partner in developing a relationship where thoughts, feelings, and concerns are discussed openly and comfortably.

Sexual function

Learning about sexual options

To help your patient with a neurologic disorder thoroughly enjoy sexual experiences, you'll need to make him aware of sexual possibilities. Encourage your patient to let his sexual partner know what his needs are. That's the only way she'll know what he likes and doesn't like. For example, tell your patient to let his partner know what he can move, areas where he has no feeling, and areas where he's sensitive to touch.

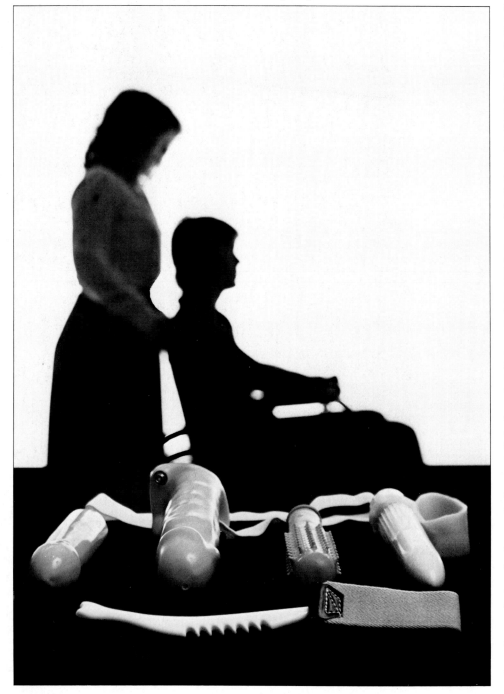

Explain to your patient that regardless of his disorder, he may still be able to use his hands, eyes, tongue, as well as conversation, imagination, and mechanical aids to increase sexual enjoyment. Tell him these sexual options will help provide intimacy, participation, and personal satisfaction.

Here are some important points to review with your patient:
• If your patient has functional use of his hands, tell him he can use his hands to sexually stimulate, or even satisfy his partner. Suggest he try body massage to find out areas which are most sexually stimulating to his partner.
• If your patient doesn't have functional use of his hands, suggest oral sexual options involving sucking, nibbling, and tongue stimulation of each other's bodies. Remind him that oral stimulation can be sexually satisfying.
• Because of your patient's physical limitations, recommend experimenting with sexual positions; for example, man on top of woman; woman on top of man; woman sitting on partner's lap facing him, and both moving in a rocking motion; anal intercourse; woman in crawling position with partner entering her from the back; and man and woman lying sideways, face to face.
• If your patient has a catheter, remind him that it's not always necessary to remove it before intercourse. After the penis is erect, the catheter may be bent and folded along the penile shaft. If your patient's female, the catheter can be pushed aside and positioned out of the way.
• If your patient has an ostomy, recommend he empty the pouch before sexual intercourse. Your patient may also want to use a pouch cover.
• If your patient's female, and has vaginal lubrication difficulties, suggest she use a water-soluble lubricant, such as K-Y Brand Lubricating Jelly.
• To get better motion during sexual activity, recommend the patient and partner consider a water bed. Another way to achieve better movement is to take advantage of muscle spasms.

If your patient has paraplegia, quadraplegia, or is not always capable of maintaining an erection, familiarize the patient with some of the mechanical aids shown in the photo at left.
• The penis stiffener (far left) is usually made of a formed piece of hard rubber that fits over the patient's penis and holds it erect for penetration.
• The dildo (second from left) is an artificial penis, usually made of semi-hard rubber, that is strapped on or above the penis. A dildo can also be hand-held.
• The vibrator (far right) is an artificial penis made of hard plastic. It is battery-operated and is hand-held.
• The flexible rubber sheath (second from right) can be placed over the vibrator for greater vaginal or anal stimulation.
• The diaphragm inserter (front) straps around the patient's wrist and aids in diaphragm insertion and removal.

Appendix

Nurses' guide to common neurologic drugs

Anticonvulsant	Anticonvulsant
Tranquilizer, respiratory depressant	
Diazepam (Valium*)	**Phenytoin sodium (Dilantin*)**

Indications and dosage

Status epilepticus; adjunctive use in convulsive disorders; tension and anxiety; skeletal muscle spasm; acute or impending delirium tremens and hallucinations; spasticity caused by upper motor neuron disorders; athetosis and tetanus
Adults: 5 to 10 mg slow I.V. push at 5 mg/minute; may repeat every 10 minutes up to maximum total dose of 30 mg.
In elderly or debilitated patients, 2 to 5 mg; may repeat every 15 minutes for two doses.
Adults and children: 2 to 10 mg P.O. b.i.d., t.i.d., or q.i.d.

Side effects

Fatigue; drowsiness; ataxia; dizziness; headache; dysarthria; slurred speech; tremor; hypotension; bradycardia; cardiovascular collapse; diplopia; blurred vision; nystagmus; nausea; constipation; change in salivation; incontinence; urinary retention; pain; phlebitis at injection site; rash; urticaria

Interactions

Phenothiazines; narcotics; barbiturates; MAO inhibitors; and other antidepressants potentiate action of diazepam (Valium*)

Precautions

• Contraindicated in shock; psychosis; coma; acute alcohol intoxication with depression of vital signs; acute narrow-angle glaucoma unless on treatment regime; and during first trimester pregnancy.
• Use cautiously in elderly or debilitated patients, and also those with limited pulmonary reserve, and in patients in whom a blood pressure drop might cause cardiovascular complications; also in patients with history of anxiety and suicidal tendencies, blood dyscrasia, hepatic or renal damage, open-angle glaucoma, and alcoholism.

Nursing considerations

• Monitor respirations every 5 to 15 minutes and before each dose repeated I.V. Have emergency resuscitative equipment and oxygen at bedside.
• To avoid phlebitis at injection site: Give I.V. slowly at rate not exceeding 5 mg/minute.
• Avoid extravasation. Do not inject I.V. using small veins.
• Do not dilute with solutions or mix with other drugs due to incompatibility.
• Drug should not be discontinued abruptly. If drug is discontinued, observe for convulsions, tremors, abdominal and muscle cramps, vomiting and sweating.
• Warn patient to avoid any activities that require alertness and good psychomotor coordination until response to drug is determined.

Indications and dosage

Grand mal, psychomotor seizures, and nonepileptic seizures following head trauma or Reye's syndrome; prevention and control of seizures during neurosurgery and status epilepticus of the grand mal type
Adults: 300 mg P.O. daily, t.i.d. or q.i.d. *Note:* This dosage may be referred to as a maintenance dose.
Loading dose
A loading dose is given if patient has not taken phenytoin sodium (Dilantin*) in the past or has a low serum level.
Adults: 900 mg to 1.5 g I.V. at 50 mg/min. divided into three doses. Do not exceed 500 mg each dose.
If patient has been receiving phenytoin sodium (Dilantin*) but has missed one or more doses and has subtherapeutic serum level. *Note:* therapeutic serum level is 10-20 mcg/ml
Adults: 100 to 300 mg I.V. at 50 mg/min.
Neuritic pain (migraine, trigeminal neuralgia, Bell's palsy)
Adults: 200 to 400 mg P.O. daily.

Side effects

Ataxia; slurred speech; confusion; dizziness; insomnia; nervousness; twitching; headache; thrombocytopenia; leukopenia; agranulocytosis; pancytopenia; macrocytosis; megaloblastic anemia; hypotension; ventricular fibrillation; nystagmus; diplopia; blurred vision; nausea; vomiting; gingival hyperplasia (especially children); toxic hepatitis; scarlet fever or measles-like rash; bullous, exfoliative or purpuric dermatitis; lupus erythematosus; hirsutism; toxic epidermal necrolysis; pain, necrosis, and inflammation at injection site; periarteritis nodosa; lymphadenopathy; hyperglycemia; osteomalacia; hypertrichosis

Interactions

• Alcohol; folic acid (Folvite*); loxapine succinate (Daxolin): cause *decreased* phenytoin sodium (Dilantin*) activity.
• Oral anticoagulants; antihistamines; chloramphenicol; diazepam (Valium*); diazoxide (Hyperstat*); disulfiram (Antabuse*); isoniazid (Hyzyd); phenylbutazone (Butazolidin*); phenyramidol; salicylates; sulfamethizole (Sulfasol); valproate sodium (Depakene Syrup): cause *increased* phenytoin sodium (Dilantin*) activity and toxicity.
• Tricyclic antidepressants in high doses may precipitate seizures, necessitating dosage adjustment.

Precautions

• Contraindicated in phenacemide (Phenurone) or hydantoin hypersensitivity; bradycardia; sinoatrial (SA) and atrioventricular (AV) node block; Stokes-Adams syndrome.
• Use cautiously in hepatic or renal dysfunction; elderly or debilitated patients; hypotension; myocardial insufficiency; respiratory depression; patients receiving other hydantoin derivatives.

Nursing considerations

• If side effects develop, notify doctor immediately. Never stop drug suddenly.
• Instruct patient to avoid activities that require alertness and good psychomotor coordination until response to drug is determined.
• If administering parenterally: never use a cloudy solution; give direct I.V. push (flush tube with 5 ml normal saline solution before and after drug administration); if unable to give direct I.V. push, mix with normal saline solution at a concentration of 100 mg/20 ml and give over 10 minute period using a separate I.V. administration set; don't mix with 5% dextrose in water, as crystallization occurs.
• Avoid I.M. route of administration as drug may precipitate at injection site, causing tissue necrosis, and pain. I.M. route and dosage will also cause erratic blood levels.
• Warn patient that drug may discolor urine pink or red, to reddish brown.
• Instruct patient to take medication at the prescribed times.
• Tell patient to carry identification stating that he's taking phenytoin sodium (Dilantin*).
• Stress importance of good oral hygiene and regular dental exams to minimize gingival hyperplasia.

*Available in both the United States and in Canada

Appendix

Nurses' guide to common neurologic drugs continued

Corticosteroid	Diuretic	Histamine receptor antagonist

Dexamethasone (Decadron*)

Indications and dosage
Cerebral edema
Adults: Initially, 10 mg (phosphate) I.V. then 4 to 6 mg I.V. or I.M. every 6 hours for 2 to 4 days; then decrease dosage over 5 to 7 days.
Inflammatory conditions, allergic reactions, neoplasia
Adults: 0.25 to 4 mg P.O. b.i.d., t.i.d, or q.i.d. or 4 to 16 mg (acetate) I.M. into joint or soft tissue every 1 to 3 weeks; or 0.8 to 1.6 mg (acetate) into lesions every 1 to 3 weeks.

Side effects
Euphoria; insomnia; psychotic behavior; congenital heart failure; hypertension; edema; cataracts; glaucoma; increased intraocular pressure; peptic ulcer; GI irritation; increased appetite; severe hypokalemia; hyperglycemia; and carbohydrate intolerance; glycosuria; impaired wound healing; various skin eruptions, including acne; muscle weakness; pancreatitis; hirsutism; and susceptibility to infections. Acute adrenal insufficiency may follow increased stress (such as infection, surgery, trauma) or abrupt withdrawal after long-term therapy
Note: Most side effects of corticosteroids are dose- or duration-related.
Withdrawal symptoms: rebound inflammation; fatigue; weakness; arthralgia; fever; dizziness; lethargy; depression; fainting; orthostatic hypotension; dyspnea; anorexia; and hypoglycemia

Interactions
• Barbiturates, phenytoin sodium (Dilantin*), and rifampin (Rifadin*) cause *decreased* corticosteroid effect.
• Indomethacin (Indocin), and aspirin (A.S.A.): cause *increased risk* of GI distress and bleeding. Administer dexamethasone (Decadron*) cautiously when patient is also receiving indomethacin (Indocin) and aspirin (A.S.A.).

Precautions
• Contraindicated in systemic fungal infections, and for alternate-day therapy.
• Use cautiously in GI ulceration or renal disease; hypertension; osteoporosis; varicella; vaccinia; exanthem; diabetes mellitus; Cushing's syndrome; thromboembolic disorders; seizures; myasthenia gravis; metastatic cancer; congestive heart failure; tuberculosis; ocular herpes simplex; hypoalbuminemia; and emotional instability or psychotic tendencies.
• *Sudden withdrawal may be fatal.*

Nursing considerations
• Give I.M. injection deep into gluteal muscle. Avoid subcutaneous administration, as atrophy and sterile abscesses may occur.
• Monitor patient's weight, blood pressure, and serum electrolyte and serum glucose levels.
• Inspect patient's skin for petechiae. Warn patient that he will bruise easily.
• Instruct patient to carry a card indicating his need for supplemental systemic glucocorticoids during stress, especially as dose is decreased.
• Tell patient not to discontinue drug abruptly without doctor's consent.
• Teach patient signs of early adrenal insufficiency; for example, fatigue, muscle weakness, and joint pain.

Mannitol (Osmitrol*)

Indications and dosage
Edema
100 g as a 10% to 20% solution over 2 to 6 hour period.
To reduce intraocular pressure or intracranial pressure (ICP)
1.5 to 2 g/Kg as a 20% to 25% solution I.V. over 30 to 60 minutes.

Side effects
Rebound increase in ICP 8 to 12 hours after diuresis; transient expansion of plasma volume during infusion, causing circulatory overload and pulmonary edema; headache; confusion; tachycardia; angina-like chest pain; blurred vision; rhinitis; thirst; nausea; vomiting; urinary retention; fluid and electrolyte imbalances; water intoxication; cellular dehydration

Interactions
None significant

Precautions
• Contraindicated in anuria; severe pulmonary congestion; pulmonary edema; severe congestive heart disease; severe dehydration; metabolic edema; progressive renal disease or dysfunction; progressive heart failure during administration; active intracranial bleeding, except during craniotomy.

Nursing considerations
• Monitor vital signs, including central venous pressure (CVP), and intake/output, hourly (report increasing oliguria).
• Monitor daily weights, renal function, fluid balance, and serum electrolytes including serum osmolality level.
• During diuretic therapy to reduce intracranial pressure, alternate drug with furosemide (Lasix*), as ordered.
• Administer infusions I.V. via an in-line filter.
• Solution may crystallize, especially at low temperatures. To redissolve, warm bottle in hot water bath, and shake it vigorously. Cool to body temperature before administering. Do not use solution with undissolved crystals.
• Give frequent mouth care or fluids to relieve thirst.
• Observe I.V. site for signs and symptoms of infiltration, such as: inflammation, edema, and potential necrosis.

Cimetidine (Tagamet*)

Indications and dosage
Duodenal ulcer prophylaxis
Adults and children over 16 years: 300 mg I.V. or P.O. every 6 hours. Maximum daily dose is 2,400 mg.

Side effects
Confusion; dizziness; mild and transient diarrhea; perforation of chronic peptic ulcers after abrupt cessation of drug; interstitial nephritis; transient elevations in blood urea nitrogen (BUN) and serum creatinine levels; jaundice; acne-like rash; urticaria; exfoliative dermatitis; hypersensitivity; muscle pain; reduced sperm count; mild gynecomastia after use longer than 1 month (but with no change in endocrine function)

Interactions
• Antacids may interfere with drug absorption. Allow 1 hour between administration of cimetidine (Tagamet*) and antacids.
• Warfarin-type anticoagulants potentiated by cimetidine (Tagamet*). Monitor prothrombin time closely.
• Antimetabolites and alkylating agents administered with drug will cause a decrease in white blood cells, and agranulocytosis.

Precautions
• Elderly patients are more susceptible to cimetidine-induced confusion. Doses should be decreased in elderly patients and in patients with renal insufficiency.
• Symptomatic response to drug therapy does not rule out possibility of a malignant gastric tumor.
• Large parenteral doses should be avoided in asthmatic patients.

Nursing considerations
• I.M. route of administration is contraindicated.
• Administer with meals to maintain blood levels.
• Hemodialysis reduces blood level of cimetidine (Tagamet*). Schedule cimetidine dose at end of hemodialysis treatment.
• I.V. solutions compatible for dilution are: normal saline solution, 5% and 10% dextrose (and combinations of these), lactated Ringer's solution and 5% sodium bicarbonate injection.
• Do not dilute medication with sterile water for injection.
• Slightly elevated serum creatinine levels may be observed.

*Available in both the United States and in Canada

Acknowledgements

Analgesic	Analgesic
Narcotic	**Nonnarcotic, antipyretic**
Codeine (sulfate, phosphate)	**Acetaminophen (Tylenol*)**

Indications and dosage
Mild to moderate pain
Adults: 15 to 60 mg P.O. or 15 to 60 mg (phosphate) subcutaneous or I.M. every 4 hours, as needed.

Side effects
Sedation; clouded sensorium; euphoria; convulsions (with large doses); hypotension, bradycardia; nausea; vomiting; constipation; ileus; urinary retention; respiratory depression; physical dependence

Interactions
General anesthetics; other narcotic analgesics; tranquilizers; sedatives; hypnotics; alcohol; tricyclic antidepressants; MAO inhibitors

Precautions
Use with extreme caution in patients with head injuries; increased intracranial pressure; increased cerebrospinal fluid pressure; severe central nervous system depression; respiratory depression; hepatic or renal disease; hypothyroidism; Addison's disease; acute alcoholism; seizures; chronic obstructive pulmonary disease (COPD); shock; or in elderly or debilitated patients.

Nursing considerations
• Use cautiously—analgesics will cause increased central nervous system (CNS) depression.
• For full analgesic effect, give before patient has intense pain.
• To potentiate effect of codeine sulfate, administer with aspirin (A.S.A.) or acetaminophen (Tylenol*).
• Do not administer discolored injection solution.
• Monitor respiratory and circulatory status, including urine output and bowel function.
• Instruct ambulatory patients that codeine sulfate causes drowsiness, and they should avoid activities that require alertness and good psychomotor coordination, such as driving a vehicle.

Indications and dosage
Mild pain or fever
Adults and children over 10 years: 325 to 600 mg P.O. or rectally every 4 hours, as needed. Maximum 2.6 g daily.

Side effects
Severe liver toxicosis with massive doses; rash; urticaria

Interactions
None significant

Precautions
High doses or unsupervised chronic use can cause liver damage. Excessive ingestion of alcoholic beverages may enhance liver toxicosis.

Nursing considerations
Administer acetaminophen (Tylenol*) to patients allergic to or unable to tolerate aspirin (A.S.A.). *Note:* acetaminophen has no anti-inflammatory effect.

We'd like to thank the following people and companies for their help with this PHOTOBOOK:

AACOMED HOSPITAL EQUIPMENT & SUPPLIES
Philadelphia, Pa.
Harry Weiler, Manager

ACCURATE MEDICAL SERVICE
Willow Grove, Pa.
Chuck Hepler, Manager

ACME UNITED CORPORATION
Medical Products Division
Bridgeport, Conn.
James F. Farrington
Senior Vice President, Marketing

AMERICAN PHARMASEAL
Glendale, Calif.
Dale Bermond, Market Manager
Diagnostic Products

CINCINNATI SUB-ZERO PRODUCTS, INC.
Cincinnati, Ohio

CONCEPT, INC.
Clearwater, Fla.

KINETIC CONCEPTS, INC.
San Antonio, Tex.

MARION LABORATORIES, INC.
Kansas City, Mo.

PURITAN-BENNETT CORPORATION
Bellmawr, N.J.

J. SKLAR MFG. CO., INC.
Long Island City, N.Y.

STRYKER CORPORATION
Kalamazoo, Mich.

SUPPORT SYSTEMS INTERNATIONAL INC.
Johns Island, S.C.

TECA CORPORATION
Pleasantville, N.Y.

Also the staffs of:

ALBERT EINSTEIN MEDICAL CENTER
Northern Division
Philadelphia, Pa.

ALLENTOWN AND SACRED HEART HOSPITAL CENTER
Allentown, Pa.

BERKS COUNTY VISITING NURSE SERVICE
Reading, Pa.

CHESTNUT HILL HOSPITAL
Philadelphia, Pa.

COMMUNITY GENERAL HOSPITAL
Reading, Pa.

DOYLESTOWN HOSPITAL
Doylestown, Pa.

EPISCOPAL HOSPITAL
Philadelphia, Pa.

FLEETWOOD VOLUNTEER AMBULANCE CORPS
Fleetwood, Pa.

THOMAS JEFFERSON UNIVERSITY HOSPITAL
Philadelphia, Pa.

WARMINSTER GENERAL HOSPITAL
Warminster, Pa.

*Available in both the United States and in Canada

Selected references

Books

Adams, Raymond D., and Maurice Victor. PRINCIPLES OF NEUROLOGY. New York: McGraw-Hill Book Co., 1977.

Armstrong, M., et al. McGRAW-HILL'S HANDBOOK OF CLINICAL NURSING. New York: McGraw-Hill Book Co., 1979.

Bannister, Roger, ed. BRAIN'S CLINICAL NEUROLOGY, 5th ed. New York: Oxford University Press, 1978.

Becker, Elle F. FEMALE SEXUALITY FOLLOWING SPINAL CORD INJURY. Bloomington, Ill.: Cheever Publishing, Inc., 1978.

Boston Women's Health Book Collective. OUR BODIES, OURSELVES, 2nd ed. New York: Simon and Schuster, Inc., 1976.

Bregman, Sue. SEXUALITY AND THE SPINAL CORD INJURED WOMAN. Minneapolis, Minn.: Sister Kenny Institute, 1975.

Brunner, Lillian S. THE LIPPINCOTT MANUAL OF NURSING PRACTICE, 2nd ed. Philadelphia: J.B. Lippincott Co., 1978.

Brunner, Lillian S., and Doris S. Suddarth. TEXTBOOK OF MEDICAL-SURGICAL NURSING, 4th ed. Philadelphia: J.B. Lippincott Co., 1980.

Chusid, Joseph G. CORRELATIVE NEUROANATOMY AND FUNCTIONAL NEUROLOGY, 17th ed. Los Altos, Calif.: Lange Medical Publications, 1979.

Clark, Ronald G., ed. MANTHER AND GATZ'S ESSENTIALS OF CLINICAL NEUROANATOMY AND NEUROPHYSIOLOGY, 5th ed. Philadelphia: F.A. Davis Co., 1975.

Comfort, Alex. A GOOD AGE. New York: Simon and Schuster, Inc., 1978.

Conway, Barbara L. CARINI AND OWENS' NEUROLOGICAL AND NEUROSURGICAL NURSING, 7th ed. St. Louis: C.V. Mosby Co., 1978.

COPING WITH NEUROLOGIC PROBLEMS PROFICIENTLY. Nursing Skillbook® Series. Springhouse, Pa.: Intermed Communications, Inc., 1981.

Davis, Joan E., and Celestine B. Mason. NEUROLOGIC CRITICAL CARE. New York: Van Nostrand Reinhold Co., 1979.

Goldberg, Stephen. CLINICAL NEUROANATOMY MADE RIDICULOUSLY SIMPLE. Miami: MedMaster, Inc., 1979.

Green, Richard. HUMAN SEXUALITY, 2nd ed. Baltimore: Williams and Wilkins Co., 1979.

Heilman, Kenneth M., et al. HANDBOOK FOR DIFFERENTIAL DIAGNOSIS OF NEUROLOGIC SIGNS AND SYMPTOMS. New York: Appleton-Century-Crofts, 1977.

Howe, James R. PATIENT CARE IN NEUROSURGERY. Boston: Little, Brown and Co., 1977.

Kolodny, Robert C., et al. TEXTBOOK OF SEXUAL MEDICINE. Boston: Little, Brown and Co., 1979.

Lewis, Edith P., and Mary H. Browning. NURSE IN COMMUNITY HEALTH. New York: American Journal of Nursing Co., 1972.

Litel, Gerald R. NEUROSURGERY AND THE CLINICAL TEAM: A GUIDE FOR NURSES, TECHNICIANS, AND STUDENTS. New York: Springer Publishing Co., Inc., 1980.

Luckmann, Joan, and Karen C. Sorenson. MEDICAL-SURGICAL NURSING: A PSYCHOPHYSIOLOGIC APPROACH, 2nd ed. Philadelphia: W.B. Saunders Co., 1980.

McConnell, James V. UNDERSTANDING HUMAN BEHAVIOR, 3rd ed. New York: Holt, Reinhart and Winston, Inc.,1980.

Merritt, H. Houston, ed. A TEXTBOOK OF NEUROLOGY, 6th ed. Philadelphia: Lea and Febiger, 1979.

Miller, Benjamin F., and Claire B. Keane. ENCYCLOPEDIA AND DICTIONARY OF MEDICINE AND NURSING. Philadelphia: W.B. Saunders Co., 1972.

Mooney, Thomas O., et al. SEXUAL OPTIONS FOR PARAPLEGICS AND QUADRIPLEGICS. Boston: Little, Brown and Co., 1975.

Oaks, Wilbur, and Gerald Melchiode, eds. SEX AND THE LIFE CYCLE. New York: Grune and Stratton, 1976.

Omer, George E., and Morton Spinner. MANAGEMENT OF PERIPHERAL NERVE PROBLEMS. Philadelphia: W. B. Saunders Co., 1980.

Osborn, Anne G. AN INTRODUCTION TO CEREBRAL ANGIOGRAPHY. New York: Harper and Row Pubs., Inc., 1980.

Plum, Fred, and Jerome Posner. THE DIAGNOSIS OF STUPOR AND COMA, 3rd ed. Philadelphia: F.A. Davis Co., 1980.

Potter, John M. THE PRACTICAL MANAGEMENT OF HEAD INJURIES, 3rd ed. Chicago: Year Book Medical Publishers, Inc. 1974.

PROVIDING EARLY MOBILITY. Nursing Photobook™ Series. Springhouse, Pa.: Intermed Communications, Inc., 1981.

Shaul, Susan, et al. TASK FORCE ON CONCERNS OF PHYSICALLY DISABLED WOMEN: WITHIN REACH. New York: Human Sciences Press, Inc., 1978.

Simpson, John F., and Kenneth R. Magee. CLINICAL EVALUATION OF THE NERVOUS SYSTEM. Boston: Little, Brown and Co., 1973.

Smith, Dorothy, and Carol P. Germain. CARE OF THE ADULT PATIENT. Philadelphia: J.B. Lippincott Co., 1975.

Snell, Richard. CLINICAL NEUROANATOMY FOR MEDICAL STUDENTS. Boston: Little, Brown and Co., 1980.

Suchenwirth, Richard. POCKET BOOK OF CLINICAL NEUROLOGY, 2nd ed. Chicago: Year Book Medical Publishers, Inc., 1979.

Sunderland, Sydney. NERVES AND NERVE INJURIES, 2nd ed. New York: Churchill-Livingston, Inc., 1979.

Swift, Nancy, and Robert M. Mabel. MANUAL OF NEUROLOGICAL NURSING. Boston: Little, Brown and Co., 1978.

Taylor, Joyce, and Sally Ballenger. NEUROLOGICAL DYSFUNCTION AND NURSING INTERVENTIONS. New York: McGraw-Hill Book Co., 1980.

Tucker, Susan M., et al. PATIENT CARE STANDARDS, 2nd ed. St. Louis: C.V. Mosby Co., 1980.

Walton, John N. ESSENTIALS OF NEUROLOGY, 4th ed. Philadelphia: J.B. Lippincott Co., 1975.

Woods, Nancy F. HUMAN SEXUALITY IN HEALTH AND ILLNESS, 2nd ed. St. Louis: C.V. Mosby Co., 1979.

Periodicals

Benedek, Laura. *The Psycho-Social Problems of Neurosurgery Patients and Their Families,* JOURNAL OF NEUROSURGICAL NURSING, 5:10-14, July 1973.

Blount, M., et al. *Symposium on Care of the Patient with Neuromuscular Disease: Management of the Patient with Amyotrophic Lateral Sclerosis,* NURSING CLINICS OF NORTH AMERICA, 14:157-171, March 1979.

Griggs, Wiwona. *Staying Well While Growing Old: Sex and the Elderly,* AMERICAN JOURNAL OF NURSING, 78:1352-1354, August 1978.

Hodges, Linda C. *Human Sexuality and the Spinal Cord Injured: Role of the Clinical Nurse Specialist,* JOURNAL OF NEUROSURGICAL NURSING, 10:125-129, September 1978.

Kavchak-Keyes, Maryanne. *Autonomic Hyperreflexia,* ARN JOURNAL, 2:17-21, September-October 1977.

Parkinson, J. *The Spinal Cord Injured Patient: Autonomic Hyperreflexia,* JOURNAL OF NEUROSURGICAL NURSING, 9:1-4, March 1977.

Piotrowski, Marcia M. *Functioning of the Normal and Neurogenic Bladder,* ARN JOURNAL, 5:13-20, March-April 1980.

Rimel, R.W., and G.W. Tyson. *The Neurologic Examination in Patients with Central Nervous System Trauma,* JOURNAL OF NEUROSURGICAL NURSING, 11:148-155, September 1979.

Romano, Mary D. *Sexual Forum: Sex and the Handicapped,* NURSING CARE, 10:18-20, July 1977.

Teasdale, G., et al. *Acute Impairment of Brain Function: Assessing Consciousness Levels,* NURSING TIMES, 71:914-917, June 12, 1975.

Teasdale G., et al. *Acute Impairment of Brain Function: Observation Record Chart,* NURSING TIMES, 71:972-973, June 19, 1975.

Williamson-Kirkland, Thomas E., and Rosemarian Berni. *Neurological Aspects of Rehabilitation: Brain Injury,* ARN JOURNAL, 5:10-12, May-June 1980.

Williamson-Kirkland, Thomas E., and Rosemarian Berni. *Neurological Aspects of Rehabilitation: Spinal Cord Injury...The Urological, Sexual and Bowel Deficits Which Result,* ARN JOURNAL, 5:8-12, July-August 1980.

Index

Index